The Neurology Riddle Book

Series Authors
Dr James Dolbow
University Hospitals Cleveland Medical Center, Cleveland, Ohio, USA

Dr Neel Fotedar
University Hospitals Cleveland Medical Center, Cleveland, Ohio, USA

Dr Joshua Edmondson
University Hospitals Cleveland Medical Center, Cleveland, Ohio, USA

Also in this series:
The Neuroanatomy Riddle Book: 150 Fun and Challenging
Neuroanatomy Riddles
James Dolbow, Joshua Edmondson, Neel Fotedar
ISBN 9781009527415

The Neurology Riddle Book

150 Common and Rare Neurological Diseases in Riddle Form

James Dolbow

University Hospitals Cleveland Medical Center

Neel Fotedar

University Hospitals Cleveland Medical Center

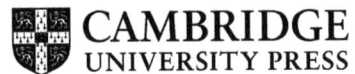

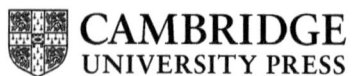

CAMBRIDGE
UNIVERSITY PRESS

Shaftesbury Road, Cambridge CB2 8EA, United Kingdom

One Liberty Plaza, 20th Floor, New York, NY 10006, USA

477 Williamstown Road, Port Melbourne, VIC 3207, Australia

314–321, 3rd Floor, Plot 3, Splendor Forum, Jasola District Centre, New Delhi – 110025, India

103 Penang Road, #05–06/07, Visioncrest Commercial, Singapore 238467

Cambridge University Press is part of Cambridge University Press & Assessment, a department of the University of Cambridge.

We share the University's mission to contribute to society through the pursuit of education, learning and research at the highest international levels of excellence.

www.cambridge.org
Information on this title: www.cambridge.org/9781009527361

DOI: 10.1017/9781009527378

© James Dolbow and Neel Fotedar 2025

First published 2025

A catalogue record for this publication is available from the British Library

Library of Congress Cataloging-in-Publication Data
Names: Dolbow, James, author. | Fotedar, Neel, author.
Title: The neurology riddle book : 150 common and rare neurological diseases in riddle form / James Dolbow, University Hospitals Cleveland Medical Center, Neel Fotedar, University Hospitals Cleveland Medical Center.
Description: Cambridge, United Kingdom ; New York, NY : Cambridge University Press, 2024. | Includes index.
Identifiers: LCCN 2024010726 (print) | LCCN 2024010727 (ebook) | ISBN 9781009527361 (paperback) | ISBN 9781009527378 (epub)
Subjects: LCSH: Neurology-Miscellanea. | Neurology-Humor. | Riddles.
Classification: LCC RC346 .D65 2024 (print) | LCC RC346 (ebook) | DDC 616.8002/07–dc23/eng/20240408
LC record available at https://lccn.loc.gov/2024010726
LC ebook record available at https://lccn.loc.gov/2024010727

ISBN 978-1-009-52736-1 Paperback

. . . .

This book is dedicated to our patients.

Contents

Foreword   viii
Zachary London
Preface   xi

Riddles and Answers 1–150   1

Index   471

Foreword

All my favorite seasonal traditions take place in October. We set up an eight-foot inflatable spider in the front yard, slice up a few pumpkins, and snuggle in front of our favorite horror films. And yes, I contend that candy corn is the ambrosia of the gods, and I will fight anyone who says otherwise.

My October reading list is also seasonal, but it falls into an entirely different genre. You see, autumn is when medical students apply for neurology residency positions, so after we finish watching "Cabin in the Woods" for the sixth time, I get to settle down in bed with a hefty stack of personal statements from aspiring neurologists.

Slasher flicks lean heavily on classic movie tropes ... creepy clowns, cars that will not start, victims deciding to split up for no reason. Similarly, the neurology personal statement depends on charmingly predictable devices and common themes. If you want to write a personal statement that incorporates every trope, try this:

Paragraph 1: I value patients as people.

Paragraph 2: My colleagues say there are no treatments for neurologic diseases, but they are categorically wrong! We can treat anything! (This paragraph must include several exclamation points.)

Paragraph 3: I'll never forget the deeply impactful moments when my parents read to me the collected works of Oliver Sacks while I was in utero.

Paragraph 4: I witnessed firsthand the devastating effects of neurologic illness on my beloved distant relative. (Note: If I am also applying to urology, I have a modified version of this paragraph in which my distant relative is devastated by an enlarged prostate.)

Paragraph 5: My greatest desire is to incorporate research into my career. Or at least, I assume that's what you want to hear, so I'm saying it.

Paragraph 6: I LOVE PUZZLES.

This last paragraph is by far the most universal. Neurologists-to-be cannot get enough puzzles. For some it is jigsaw puzzles, Rubik's cubes, and escape rooms. Others fancy themselves the next Sherlock Holmes, Miss Marple, or Hercule Poirot. One applicant pointed out that Batman was known as The World's Greatest Detective before he was The Caped Crusader.

And while I'm callously teasing these poor medical students right now, they are not wrong. Most of us were drawn to neurology in part because we genuinely love a good brain teaser. Neurology is not the only diagnostic field, but our reliance on overlapping neuroanatomic pathways to localize lesions is unique in medicine. And even when cases are more about pattern recognition than localization, we rely on an amalgam of subtle clues from the history and examination to reach a verdict. A good detective story is full of details, and that, my friends, is why our notes are so maddeningly long.

And so all you Nancy Drews and Batmen have a hard-to-reach diagnostic itch to scratch. But fear not! With *The Neurology Riddle Book*, James Dolbow and Neel Fotedar have created a long-armed backscratcher that will hit the spot perfectly. The book you are holding is just dripping with intensely satisfying rhyming puzzles, guaranteed to probe your knowledge of neurologic illnesses from common to... (spoiler alert) Fatal Familial Insomnia.

One of the reasons I'm most excited about "*The Neurology Riddle Book,*" is that it is full of delicious rhyming couplets. Neurology has a storied history of educational rhymes, dating back to 1859 when Swiss ophthalmologist Johann Horner threw his penlight across the room with excitement upon discovering the mnemonic brilliance of "Ptosis, miosis, and anhidrosis." This was followed by "C3, 4, 5 keep the diaphragm alive," "First, worst, or cursed," and the novel sodium-themed rhyme, "High to low, your brain will blow. Low to high, your pons will fry."

With "*The Neurology Riddle Book*" and its predecessor, "*The Neuroanatomy Riddle Book*," the number of canonical neurology rhymes has ballooned from 4 to 304. Arguably, this is a historically significant scientific achievement that has taken place in our lifetimes. It's the kind of exciting progress in our field that will inspire future generations, and I look forward to reading more about it in the final paragraphs of neurology personal statements next October.

Zach London, M.D.

Preface

If you love neuroscience, especially neurology, chances are you love a good puzzle. This book aims to provide readers, from medical students to experienced neurologists, with fun and challenging riddles about clinical neurology. It includes 150 four-line riddles describing specific high-yield neurological syndromes, conditions, and diseases in cryptic form.

Answers can be any of the following:

1. A neurodegenerative disease
2. A movement disorder
3. A stroke type or neurological vascular event
4. A seizure disorder
5. A neuroimmunological condition
6. A neuroinfectious disease
7. A sleep disorder
8. A neuromuscular/myopathic disease

All riddles will include hints to help you identify the condition such as patient demographic, clinical presentation, or underlying pathophysiology, and if you are still stumped by the end of the riddle, at the bottom of the page you will find two additional hints to help guide you. On the following page, you will find the answer to the riddle along with a complete description of the condition, including the history of the disease, pathophysiology, clinical presentation, diagnostics, treatment, and prognosis.

Enjoy!

1

• • • • •

From bleed outside of brain,
Crescent-shaped, from tear in vein,
Can cause shift, and cross bone lines,
And on CT, see bright it shines.

Hint #1

The answer is in your potential space.

Hint #2

Do not falsely localize the wrong answer.

Subdural Hematoma

Characterized by blood in the potential space between the arachnoid membrane and the dura mater, subdural hematomas are most commonly caused by the tearing of bridging veins as a result of brain movement within the skull. These veins drain from the brain surface into the dural venous sinuses. The elderly and individuals with alcoholism are most prone to developing subdural hematoma.

Subdural hematomas can occur both acutely and chronically, each with significantly different clinical presentations. Acute subdural hematoma often occurs after acute closed-head trauma and by definition becomes symptomatic within 72 hours. These patients often present with severe headache and acute alterations in consciousness. Depending upon the size and location of the subdural hematoma, patients could exhibit a variety of presentations on neurological examination. For example, a patient with a large subdural hematoma over the lateral convexity of the dominant hemisphere would most likely have contralateral hemiparesis, aphasia, and ipsilateral gaze deviation.

These signs are a result of underlying cerebral edema, caused by the subdural hematoma. Clinically, this presentation can be easily confused with an acute dominant hemispheric infarction in the middle cerebral artery territory. A carefully documented history of preceding head trauma, in addition to a CT scan, and severe headache can often differentiate between the two.

In severe cases, where the edema is severe enough to compress the ipsilateral oculomotor nerve exiting the midbrain, patient will have ipsilateral pupillary dilation. However, do not be fooled as these patients can also develop uncal herniation, producing compression of the contralateral oculomotor nerve and cerebral peduncle against the tentorium. Clinically, this phenomenon, known as *Kernohan's notch phenomenon*, appears as contralateral pupillary dilation and the "falsely" localizing ipsilateral hemiparesis.

Chronic subdural hematomas more often occur in the elderly, alcoholic, and epileptic patients who are more susceptible to such injuries because of poor balance and gait issues. The relative brain atrophy of such patients puts them at a higher risk of developing subdural hematomas, even with trivial head trauma, because of the "stretching" of the bridging veins to account for the increased distance between the atrophied brain and the dura. As opposed to the predominantly focal symptomatology of acute subdural hematomas, the patients with chronic hematomas have vague and nonspecific symptoms like mild headaches, increased forgetfulness, gait ataxia, and so on. Both acute and chronic subdural hematomas can present with seizures and status epilepticus as well.

On non-contrasted CT, subdural hematomas typically appear as a crescent-shaped hyperdensity (acute) or isodensity-hypodensity (chronic) that commonly crosses suture lines. Chronic subdural hematomas are often isodense to cerebrospinal fluid (CSF) and hypodense to adjacent cortex, and hence they can be difficult to identify on a CT scan.

The treatment of acute subdural hematoma depends upon its clinical presentation and size. If the patient is on anticoagulation, reversal of the specific anticoagulant is recommended. For patients with rapidly declining consciousness, large hematoma (>10 mm), and midline shift (>5 mm), emergent neurosurgical consultation is warranted. Such patients often require emergent craniotomy with evacuation of the hematoma. The management of chronic subdural hematoma is not straightforward. Craniotomy with evacuation may be recommended for larger hematomas. Middle meningeal artery embolization is a new noninvasive treatment option available for such patients, which may decrease the likelihood of re-accumulation of the hematoma.

2

• • • • •

Not atonic when should be,
In sleep, enactments you will see,
Alpha-synuclean accrue,
Years later tremor comes in view.

Hint #1

History provided by bed partner.

Hint #2

When you find the answer, draw a rem around it.

REM Sleep Behavior Disorder

Rapid eye movement (REM) sleep behavior disorder (RBD) is characterized by loss of atonia that is normally present in REM sleep. In addition, patients often enact their dreams.

An intricate circuit in the brainstem and hypothalamus controls the switch between non-REM and REM sleep. A discrete group of neurons in rostral pons – precoeruleus (PC) and sublaterodorsal tegmental nucleus (SLD) – are REM-on neurons, and their activity is responsible for the behavioral state of REM sleep and atonia. The SLD nucleus, in particular, projects to the spinal cord and is responsible for REM atonia. The PC nucleus, on the other hand, projects to the basal forebrain and medial septal nuclei and is responsible for the characteristic electroencephalogram (EEG) findings seen in REM sleep. Experimental lesional studies in animals and pathological studies in humans and animals have shown that the clinical syndrome of RBD is associated with pathology seen in this specific region of rostral pons.

One of the most important differential diagnoses for patients with RBD is an underlying alpha-synucleinopathy, for example, idiopathic Parkinson disease, dementia with Lewy bodies (DLB), and multiple system atrophy (MSA). In fact, it is believed that RBD represents an early stage of such neurodegenerative diseases, as the pathological protein accumulation invades rostral pons.

The diagnosis of RBD is made by video-polysomnography. The pathological hallmark is RSWA (REM sleep without atonia). It is identified by monitoring for excessive muscle activity in chin electromyography (EMG) electrodes during a 30-second REM epoch.

The first-line treatment for RBD is melatonin, which can be used in doses ranging from 3 to 18 mg and a second-line treatment option is clonazepam. Treatment is usually reserved for patients who are at risk of injuring their bed partners or themselves. Safe sleeping practices must also be observed.

3

• • • • •

Axial spasms that appear,
Clustered in infants morning near,
Chaotic interictal waves,
Later change in how behaves.

Hint #1

Follow the cardinal directions.

Hint #2

No rhythm in those hips.

7

West Syndrome

West syndrome is an infantile epileptic encephalopathy syndrome, typically seen between the ages of 3 months and 1 year, consisting of the triad of infantile spasms, psychomotor deterioration, and a characteristic interictal EEG pattern known as *hypsarrhythmia*. This pattern consists of very large amplitude, irregular slow waves, superimposed on a disorganized background with multifocal spikes.

The infantile spasms, central to the diagnosis, are characterized by clusters of rapid axial contractions seen in both extension and flexion, usually symmetrical and often shortly after the infant awakens, followed by a period of distress and crying. The ictal EEG pattern associated with these spasms is a diffuse electrodecrement.

West syndrome can be caused by a multitude of severe structural and metabolic etiologies affecting the brain. Structural etiologies include malformations of cortical development (MCD) like hemimegalencephaly, cortical dysplasia, heterotopias, and so on. Tuberous sclerosis is a major cause of infantile spasms/West syndrome. About half of patients with tuberous sclerosis have infantile spasms. Adrenocorticotropic hormone (ACTH) is the first-line therapy for the treatment of infantile spasms. Vigabatrin is also considered an effective choice for the treatment of infantile spasms, especially in patients with underlying tuberous sclerosis. The response to treatment is monitored by cessation of clinical spasms and resolution of the hypsarrhythmia on EEG.

4

• • • • •

Most commonly found with bone break,
Out cold, lucid, then coma make,
Lens-shaped bright on CT head,
Does not cross lines, artery bled.

Hint #1

You'll know it when it hits you in the head.

Hint #2

Common injury location rhymes with "carry on."

Epidural Hematoma

This intracranial hematoma is characterized by bleeding into the epidural space. It is most commonly caused by a tear in one of the meningeal arteries (often the middle meningeal artery overlying the pterion). Most epidural hematomas are associated with skull trauma and fracture. The rupture of arteries produces a high-pressure hematoma that separates the dura from the skull, which often only stops growing after self-tamponade due to compression and occlusion of the ruptured vessel by the growing hematoma.

Some patients experience a period of lucidity ("lucid period") after the initial alteration of consciousness, which is then followed by a return to decreased consciousness, due to expansion of the hematoma and brain compression. The clinical presentation can be quite similar to those with acute subdural hematoma – sudden onset of severe headache with nausea/vomiting, seizures, contralateral hemiplegia, ipsilateral gaze deviation, and so on.

Epidural hematoma is identified on non-contrasted CT scan as an extra-axial hyperdense lens-shaped convexity, which does not cross skull suture lines and is seen compressing the brain parenchyma.

Most commonly, epidural hematomas develop in the middle meningeal fossa due to fracture at the pterion, which is the H-shaped suture formation of calvarium formed by the junction of parietal bone, frontal bone, greater wing of the sphenoid bone, and squamous region of the temporal bone.

Large hematomas (>30 cubic cm) with poor neurological exam on presentation warrants emergent neurosurgical consultation for potential craniotomy and hematoma evacuation. If the initial hematoma volume is small and the patient's neurological exam is stable, then close observation with frequent neurological checks is required. A repeat CT scan at 6 hours is often recommended to assess hematoma stability.

5

· · · · ·

Cannot move arms, or legs, or face,
Consciousness is full in this case,
Though some may think that they dead be,
Eyes can move and they can see.

Hint #1

The answer is communicated by eye movements.

Hint #2

Unlock the right answer.

Locked-in Syndrome (Bilateral Pons Lesion)

Locked-in syndrome is a notorious and devastating result of an extensive injury to the basis pontis (e.g., infarction or hemorrhage) that damages the bilateral descending corticospinal and corticobulbar tracts with relative sparing of the sensory pathways and critical reticular nuclei necessary for arousal.

Severe bilateral corticospinal tract injury leads to quadriplegia. Bilateral corticobulbar tract injury leads to impaired function of the lower cranial nerves, thus leading to facial diplegia, severe dysphagia, and anarthria.

These patients also have conjugate horizontal gaze palsy in both directions likely because of injury to bilateral abducens nuclei and excitatory burst neurons for horizontal gaze. Vertical gaze is spared since the excitatory burst neurons for vertical gaze are located in rostral midbrain.

Patients with locked-in syndrome could appear to be in coma because of lack of physical response to any stimulus. But these patients are aware and awake as evidenced by blinking and intact awake and sleep pattern on EEG. Such patients often respond with vertical eye movements.

Locked-in syndrome gained international recognition after the publication of *The Diving Bell and The Butterfly* (*Le Scaphandre et le Papillon*) by French journalist Jean-Dominique Bauby. This memoir, first published in 1997, describes his life before and after his pontine stroke, which produced locked-in syndrome.

6

. . . . .

Dysesthesias in the legs,
Formication, movement begs,
Cannot lay still, won't stay in bed,
If safe can try pro-dopa med.

Hint #1

The answer can usually be found at night.

Hint #2

You will lose sleep over it.

13

Restless Leg Syndrome

First described by seventeenth-century English anatomist and physician Thomas Willis, restless leg syndrome, a disorder he termed *"unquietness,"* is mainly characterized by the chronic symptoms of involuntary leg movements commonly caused by uncomfortable leg parasthesias (tingling, stretching, and crawling sensation on skin) and the uncontrollable urge to move, all of which are relieved with movement. This disorder was later more fully studied and described by twentieth-century Swedish neurologist Karl Axel Ekbom, who eventually coined the term "restless leg syndrome," though some still refer to this disorder as "Willis-Ekbom Disease."

The symptoms of restless leg syndrome are worse at night or when the patient becomes sleepy; however many patients experience these symptoms when awake but sitting or immobile for long periods of time. This often results in a significant barrier to sleep quality and mental health.

There is no clear cause for this disorder. In some patients, a clear family history can be identified, but no single genetic mutation has been identified so far. Some other common risk factors are iron deficiency, uremia, neuropathy, spinal cord disease, and so on.

Restless leg syndrome can be differentiated from nocturnal leg cramps as restless leg syndrome is rarely painful. Restless leg syndrome can also be differentiated from a similar condition called periodic limb movement disorder as, though both conditions include nocturnal movements in the legs and sometimes arms, in periodic limb movement disorder, the patient is unaware of the movements, and the limb movement most often occurs in sleep stages 1 and 2.

Though these conditions are clinically separate, approximately 80% of people with restless leg syndrome also have periodic limb movement disorder.

The clinical diagnosis of restless leg syndrome is best made by self-reported symptoms from the patient, with little utility of electrodiagnostic and polysomnographic testing, though serum chemistry and iron deficiency workup may help with clinical decision-making, and thus treatment of iron deficiency and uremia can be curative.

If patient's serum ferritin is low, iron replacement is the recommended treatment of choice. For patients with chronic persistent symptoms, first-line therapy is administration of a gabapentinoid, such as gabapentin or pregabalin. In patients with obesity or history of substance abuse, dopamine agonists, such as pramipexole or ropinirole, are recommended.

7

• • • • •

From Latin "fleeting," "Dark" in Greek,
And no symptoms like numb or weak,
With hampered flow through ophthalmic,
The lights go out, come back on quick.

Hint #1

The answer is behind the lowered curtain.

Hint #2

Usually only lasts seconds to minutes.

Amaurosis Fugax

Named from the joining of the Greek word *amaurosis*, meaning "dark," and the Latin word *fugax*, meaning "fleeting," amaurosis fugax is a clinical stroke syndrome characterized by sudden but transient partial or complete loss of monocular vision. This condition is also commonly called "transient monocular vision loss," though this description often includes a much larger differential.

Patients often describe this as "a curtain coming down" over the affected eye, resulting in a partial or full black/gray visual field. Though some report only these negative symptoms, some also report positive phenomena such as sparkling lights or scintillating scotomas, all of which usually resolve within seconds to minutes.

Amaurosis fugax is caused by transient occlusion of the central retinal artery or its branches by emboli. The central retinal artery is a branch of the ophthalmic artery, which is a branch of the internal carotid artery. A common source of emboli to the eye is the extracranial internal carotid artery. Such patients must be admitted to the hospital and must have a thorough stroke workup, including head and neck vessel imaging. This embolized cholesterol can often be seen on ophthalmologic examination of the retina (Hollenhorst plaques).

Treatment depends upon the cause. In patients with severe carotid artery stenosis, surgical treatment like endarterectomy is the treatment of choice. Patients are often placed on chronic antiplatelet therapy for secondary stroke prevention.

8

• • • • •

A stepwise change in one's mentation,
With change in strength or in sensation,
Infarcts on imaging seen,
Subcortical pattern less keen.

Hint #1

Prevention is the best treatment.

Hint #2

Binswanger might know.

Vascular Dementia

Vascular dementia is characterized by a progressive cognitive decline in patients as a result of episodic and/or progressive cerebrovascular disease. These vascular insults can come in the form of a single or multiple ischemic or hemorrhagic strokes, or ischemic white matter disease, or as a result of global cerebral hypoperfusion (seen in hypotension or cardiac arrest), as well as other hemorrhagic cerebrovascular conditions such as subdural and subarachnoid hemorrhage. The criteria for the diagnosis of vascular dementia are as follows: 1) dementia; 2) one or more cerebrovascular insults that are both clinically and radiologically evident; and 3) a temporal relationship between the cerebrovascular insults and the dementia. This typically takes place in a "stepwise" manner with a paired decline in the patient's functional and cognitive abilities.

Vascular dementia also goes by many names based on the location and types of cerebrovascular disease implicated. *Binswanger disease* refers to the cognitive decline seen in patients with small-vessel ischemic disease resulting in multiple lacunar infarcts in the basal ganglia as well as the subcortical and periventricular white matter. Intuitively, *multiple-infarct dementia* refers to the progressive cognitive decline in patients with multiple large-vessel infarcts.

Strategic-infarct dementia refers to the cognitive decline in patients with a "single infarct" in the ACA, PCA, or angular gyrus territories, producing memory impairment along with abulia/aphasia/dyspraxia, amnesia/agitation/hallucinations, or aphasia/alexia/agraphia, respectively. Bihemispheric cerebral insults are often needed to produce symptoms consistent with dementia.

Vascular dementia can clinically mimic Alzheimer's dementia. However, the early cognitive symptoms in vascular dementia are more of a "subcortical" nature such as prominent apathy, bradyphrenia, as well as impaired concentration and executive function. On the other hand, patients with Alzheimer's disease often have significant memory impairment in early stages. Additionally, in patients with bihemispheric cerebral impairment, pseudobulbar affect, so-called emotional incontinence, is not uncommon.

Given vascular dementia is a clinical diagnosis based on cognitive decline paired temporally with one or more cerebrovascular insults that are both clinically and radiologically evident, there is no confirmatory testing available and the prognosis of vascular dementia is highly variable.

The treatment in vascular dementia mainly relies on the modification of vascular risk factors and secondary stroke prevention. These include management of hypertension, diabetes, dyslipidemia, and antiplatelet or anticoagulant therapy. Cholinestrase inhibitors, such as donepezil or rivastigmine, can be used in such patients as well. These drugs are primarily used for Alzheimer's disease; however studies have shown that a significant proportion of patients with vascular dementia have coexisting Alzheimer's disease as well.

9

. . . . .

Pupil dysfunction, no vibration,
Brain involved post-chancre station,
Can have strokes if vessels in,
Corkscrews that hate penicillin.

Hint #1

Then answer is usually painless.

Hint #2

Nineteenth-century surgeon Douglas Argyll Robertson would know.

Neurosyphilis

Caused by infection with the corkscrew-shaped spirochetes *Treponemal pallidum*, neurosyphilis is often preceded by untreated primary syphilis that manifests as a painless genital ulcer or chancre. The ulcer typically heals in 3–6 weeks. The central nervous system (CNS) manifestations can develop anytime after that. However, in approximately 25% of primary syphilis cases, asymptomatic seeding of the CNS can occur, resulting in a latent infection that manifests years to decades later.

CNS manifestations of neurosyphilis include meningitis, stroke, tabes dorsalis, dementia paralytica, gummas, Charcot joints, Argyll Robertson pupils, spinal myelitis, among others. Syphilitic meningitis (early stage neurosyphilis) often presents with the typical signs of meningitis such as headache, neck stiffness, and photophobia. Additionally, ocular manifestations such as uveitis and/or retinitis and otologic manifestations such as hearing loss and tinnitus can also be seen in early neurosyphilis. Strokes can also result from meningovascular syphilis that presents as small (Nissl-Alzheimer arteritis) and medium or large (Heubner's arteritis) intracranial artery inflammation, resulting in luminal narrowing and thrombus formation.

Tabes dorsalis is a form of late (tertiary) neurosyphilis occurring in approximately 10% of untreated syphilis that results in the demyelination of the posterior columns of the spinal cord, in turn causing decreased position and vibratory sense, severe electrical-type back and leg pain, ataxia, areflexia, and bowel and bladder dysfunction.

Additionally, this condition can lead to Charcot joints due to sensory loss and subsequent joint destruction. Argyll Robertson pupils commonly exist in patients with tabes dorsalis. These pupils do not react to light but do react to accommodation (light-near dissociation).

Cerebral syphilitic gummas constitute another form of tertiary syphilis that results in the development of granulomatous mass lesions in the brain, which are a local inflammatory response, usually of the surrounding dura and enhance with contrasted MRI. Dementia paralytica, also called "general paresis" is a condition seen in chronic meningoencephalitis and often presents as mania, psychosis, and dementia.

If neurosyphilis is clinically suspected in patients without coexisting HIV, the workup should begin with serum testing like FTA-ABS (fluorescent treponemal antibody-absorbed test) or CIA (chemiluminescence immunoassay). If these tests are reactive, treatment must be initiated. If the tests are nonreactive, then the diagnosis is ruled out. In early stages of neurosyphilis with mild and nonspecific neurological symptoms, the positive serum test must be followed by CSF analysis. If the CSF VDRL test is positive, treatment must be started. If the CSF VDRL is negative, but there is a pleocytosis, treatment must be initiated. In patients with HIV and a positive serum test, if there are neurological symptoms consistent with neurosyphilis, then CSF analysis must be done. If CSF VDRL is positive, treatment must be initiated.

The CDC-approved treatment for neurosyphilis consists of aqueous crystalline penicillin G dosed 3-4 million units IV every 4 hours for 10-14 days or Procaine penicillin G dosed 2.4 million units IM with probenecid 500 mg oral 4 times a day for 10-14 days.

10

• • • • •

Crossway lesion, many cause,
Sensation level, bathroom flaws,
Hyperintense on spine T2,
LP confirm, then steroids do.

Hint #1

Increased reflexes.

Hint #2

If that does not work, consider intravenous immunoglobulin (IVIG) or plasma exchange.

Transverse Myelitis

Transverse myelitis is an inflammation of the spinal cord that commonly presents with acute to subacute bilateral motor weakness and sensation changes below the level of the spinal cord lesion, as well as anal and urinary sphincter control impairment. The causes of transverse myelitis can be viral, bacterial, parasitic, rheumatological/antibody-mediated, vascular, paraneoplastic, demyelinating, or idiopathic. Idiopathic transverse myelitis is typically a monophasic illness. Most cases of transverse myelitis are related to an underlying autoimmune condition like multiple sclerosis, neuromyelitis optica spectrum disorder (NMOSD), or myelin oligodendrocyte glycoprotein (MOG)-associated disorder.

Diagnosis of transverse myelitis requires advanced imaging of the spinal cord, most accurately with a contrasted MRI study. This also helps to rule out compressive pathology that can mimic transverse myelitis. The next step in the diagnostic workup often includes admission to the hospital and lumbar puncture for CSF analysis.

Typical MRI findings include a T2 hyperintense intramedullary signal change. Most cases also show post-Gadolinium enhancement of the lesion. If the lesion is extensive (three or more vertebral segments), it is called longitudinally extensive transverse myelitis (LETM). It is critical to recognize this pattern as it is mostly seen in patients with NMOSD.

CSF analysis typically shows pleocytosis and elevated protein. Other labs that must be checked include IgG index, oligoclonal bands, and CSF AQP-4 (aquaporin 4) antibody analysis. Serum AQP-4 and MOG antibodies must also be checked.

An MRI of the brain must also be performed in order to assess the demyelinating lesions in the brain.

Patients with acute transverse myelitis must be urgently treated with high-dose IV corticosteroids after an infectious etiology has been ruled out. Plasma exchange should be considered in patients with poor response to steroids or in cases of very extensive disease.

Patients who are likely to have an underlying disease like multiple sclerosis or NMOSD are at a higher risk of recurrence. Such patients must be treated with appropriate long-term immunotherapy.

11

• • • • •

Elevated CK's vast,
And X-linked recessively passed,
Mostly in boys and at young age,
Gower's sign, decreased calf gage.

Hint #1

Tip toe your way to the right answer.

Hint #2

Do not let the answer go the way of the dystrophin.

Duchenne Muscular Dystrophy

Duchenne muscular dystrophy is the most severe form of muscular dystrophy in children, as well as the most common. Duchenne muscular dystrophy and its milder phenotype, Becker muscular dystrophy, are called dystrophinopathies as they are caused by mutations in the gene *DMD*, which encodes for the protein dystrophin. The *DMD* gene is the largest yet identified gene in humans and is located on the short arm of the X chromosome. Dystrophin serves as a vital cytoplasmic protein that connects muscle fiber cytoskeleton to the extracellular matrix. The phenotype of the dystrophinopathy depends upon the amount of residual dystrophin protein. In the most severe phenotype, which is Duchenne muscular dystrophy, the dystrophin is either completely absent or very minimal in amount.

The absence of dystrophin results in progressive proximal muscle weakness and delayed motor milestones beginning from the age of 1–5 years. The weakness affects lower extremities before upper extremities; hence these patients are often first noticed to have more frequent falls than other children of their age. They have difficulty walking, running, jumping, and climbing up stairs. Additionally, children with Duchenne muscular dystrophy experience enlargement of their calves (pseudohypertrophy). Gower's maneuver describes a child attempting to stand from a seated position on the floor by walking their hands up their thighs in order to stand. With the progression of the disease, most of these children will require a wheelchair by age 12. Many patients will die in their 20s due to heart or respiratory failure, caused by the progressive fatty-infiltration of the heart and lungs. These children often develop a dilated cardiomyopathy along with multiple conduction abnormalities. Typical EKG findings include a negative P wave and a tall R wave in V1, along with right axis deviation.

After clinical suspicion is raised due to the multiple delayed motor milestones early in life, additional testing will show a vastly elevated CK level of 50–100x normal, and electromyography will show myopathic features. The diagnosis is confirmed with a muscle biopsy showing absent or severely reduced muscle dystrophin. Diagnosis can also be confirmed by genetic testing.

Steroids are the mainstay of treatment for Duchenne muscular dystrophy. These have been shown to improve motor function, delay loss of ambulation and cardiomyopathy, and improve survival. Novel antisense oligonucleotide (ASO) therapies like eteplirsen are also available in some countries. Eteplirsen is FDA approved, but its approval is controversial because of methodological limitations in the trial. Further confirmatory studies are pending.

Baseline cardiac evaluation with EKG, echocardiography, or cardiac MRI is recommended in all patients, including a consultation with a cardiologist. Such evaluation is often repeated on an annual basis in asymptomatic individuals.

12

• • • • •

Paralysis, poor sensory,
Pernicious or in Crohn's you'll see,
No reflexes, toes up will be,
And spinal cord post' atrophy.

Hint #1

There *B* only one answer, or 12.

Hint #2

Ask a fish tapeworm.

Subacute Combined Degeneration

Subacute combined degeneration of the spinal cord occurs in individuals deficient in vitamin B12. This deficiency predominantly affects the dorsal column pathways and the lateral corticospinal tracts. Clinically, the patients present with a subacute to chronic weakness, paresthesias, and ataxia. Over time, they can develop spasticity because of involvement of the corticospinal tracts, hence presenting as a myelopathy. As opposed to a typical myelopathy, the reflexes are often diminished or absent due to a coexisting peripheral neuropathy, but plantar responses are extensor. Overall, the most common neurological manifestation of B12 deficiency is a peripheral polyneuropathy.

B12 deficiency can result from many causes including gastric bypass surgery, Crohn disease, pernicious anemia, nitrous oxide ingestion, and fish tapeworm infestation (*Diphyllobothrium latum*). Some commonly used medications like proton pump inhibitors/H2 blockers and metformin can also cause clinically significant B12 deficiency.

This condition can be diagnosed using simple bloodwork where in addition to the subjective and objective exam findings, patients will have either a severely low or borderline low levels of vitamin B12 with elevated levels of methylmalonic acid and homocysteine.

MRI of the spinal cord is often seen to be normal, however can show atrophy or abnormal signal in the posterior portions. Patients must also have their complete blood count and RBC indices checked.

Patients with a coexisting anemia, especially macrocytic anemia must be evaluated for anti-intrinsic factor antibodies for a diagnosis of pernicious anemia.

Treatment is with long-term intramuscular vitamin B12 administration, with patients having mild symptoms making a full or near-full recovery, though patients with severe or long-term symptoms often experience incomplete recovery.

There are other rare nutritional deficiencies that can present as myelo-neuropathy and can clinically mimic subacute combined degeneration of spinal cord due to B12 deficiency. These include copper and vitamin E deficiency. These have become more common in modern times with advancement of bariatric surgery.

13

• • • • •

Pain and weakness, lesioned skin,
Answer lies biopsy in,
Anti-Mi-2 and V-sign be,
And look for malignancy.

Hint #1

Then answer is under the shawl.

Hint #2

The answer (and weakness) may be more proximal than you think.

Dermatomyositis

Dermatomyositis is an immune-mediated myopathy characterized by proximal weakness, muscle tenderness and pain, and cutaneous manifestations. Although it most often occurs on its own, it can also present as part of a more systemic condition such as mixed connective tissue disease, malignancy, or systemic sclerosis. The pathophysiology of dermatomyositis is thought to be a B-cell-mediated autoimmune attack of the endomysial layer of muscles, specifically the endothelium of the blood vessels in this layer.

On presentation, what differentiates dermatomyositis from polymyositis are the cutaneous manifestations. Patients with dermatomyositis are often found to have a heliotropic rash on their face as well as eyelid edema, dilated capillaries at the nailbeds, scaly eruptions and erythema on their knuckles (Gottron sign), joint erythema, and an erythematous rash on the shoulders and upper back (shawl sign) and upper chest and neck (V sign). The clinical diagnosis is supported by lab investigations, such as elevated CK levels. Antibody testing is helpful, with anti-Mi-2 antibodies being highly specific.

The characteristic EMG findings include the presence of myopathic units (low amplitude, short duration) with fibrillation potentials or positive sharp waves, indicative of active denervation. These findings indicate an inflammatory myopathy. Muscle biopsy will show perimysial and/or perivascular inflammatory infiltration, as well as perifascicular atrophy.

Treatment includes the usage of steroids and steroid-sparing agents like azathioprine and methotrexate. Such patients must also be screened for coexisting interstitial lung disease and underlying malignancy.

14

• • • • •

In those who drink and little eat,
And B vitamin is deplete,
Eyes cannot move and down they'll fall,
And make up what they cannot recall.

Hint #1

Answer correctly, win intravenous thiamine.

Hint #2

Two separate conditions combined to B-1, or lack thereof.

Wernicke–Korsakoff Syndrome

Wernicke–Korsakoff syndrome is a term used to describe two clinically separate syndromes, Wernicke encephalopathy and Korsakoff syndrome, which share the same cause and histopathology. Caused by a deficiency of thiamine (vitamin B1), Wernicke encephalopathy and Korsakoff syndrome are most commonly seen in individuals who have poor dietary intake or poor intestinal absorption or both. The most common patient population predisposed to this syndrome are alcoholics. In modern times, cancer patients and those who have undergone bariatric surgery are also susceptible.

Wernicke's encephalopathy is an acute encephalopathy that develops over the course of days to weeks. The symptoms of impaired mentation include decreased spontaneous speech, apathy, attention deficits, and impaired memory. Some characteristic abnormalities seen on ocular motility examination include vertical or gaze-evoked nystagmus and ophthalmoparesis.

Korsakoff syndrome is characterized by a more chronic retrograde and anterograde amnesia. These patients often confabulate during examination. By the time Korsakoff syndrome develops, the damage is irreversible.

The diagnosis of Wernicke's encephalopathy and Korsakoff syndrome is purely clinical. Any patient admitted to the hospital with encephalopathy with a known risk factor like alcoholism or cancer, or post undergoing bariatric surgery should be treated with high dose IV thiamine. For preventive purposes, if such patients are being admitted to the hospital for unrelated issues, especially hypoglycemia, thiamine supplementation must be done before glucose is administered to avoid precipitating Wernicke's encephalopathy. There is no need for performing an MRI or checking blood thiamine levels for diagnosis. Some characteristic MRI findings include T2/FLAIR hyperintensities in periaqueductal gray matter, medial thalami, and mammillary bodies.

15

• • • • •

Autoimmune or cancer cause,
And autonomic function flaws,
Calcium channel malefaction,
Proximal weak, improves with action.

Hint #1

The answer lies before the synapse.

Hint #2

Symptoms of arriving at the correct answer may include dry mouth, constipation, and impotence. Hooray!

Lambert Eaton Myasthenic Syndrome

Lambert Eaton myasthenic syndrome (LEMS) is an autoimmune disease caused by antibodies directed at presynaptic voltage-gated calcium channels (P/Q-type) that results in an overall reduced amount of acetylcholine released into the synaptic cleft at neuromuscular junctions and terminals of autonomic nerves. This syndrome is caused by a paraneoplastic process in 60% of patients, and of these patients, the most commonly associated cancer is small cell lung cancer. Compared to myasthenia gravis (MG), LEMS typically occurs in middle-aged adults.

The most prominent symptoms are generalized weakness, which is most prominent proximally, and is intermittent in nature, with the strength improving with exercise. Additionally, in contrast to signs and symptoms found in MG, the clinical presentation of LEMS often includes more prominent autonomic symptoms, such as dry mouth, impotence, and constipation. Interestingly, on exam, though tendon reflexes are often absent, they can be increased after activity of the involved tendon muscles. Patients with LEMS have less involvement of cranial nerves compared to MG patients, hence accounting for lesser prevalence of ocular and bulbar symptoms.

Diagnosis can be made using antibody testing and/or electromyography. Of individuals with Lambert Eaton myasthenic syndrome, 90% will have P/Q-type voltage-gated calcium channel antibodies, and up to 50% will have N-type voltage-gated calcium channel antibodies.

All patients with LEMS must undergo routine nerve conduction study (NCS) with a needle EMG study. Unlike MG, the compound muscle action potential (CMAP) amplitudes are usually significantly decreased in LEMS. The SNAP amplitudes are usually normal. Post-exercise facilitation of CMAP amplitudes is typical. It can also be achieved with high-frequency repetitive stimulation. Symptomatic treatment consists of 3,4-diaminopyridine, which is a K-channel blocker. Pyridostigmine can also be used.

16

• • • • •

Most often children, who seem to,
Stare off in space, lip smack and chew,
No shaking and no memory,
But spike and wave at hertz of 3.

Hint #1

Some come to the answer by hyperventilating.

Hint #2

Sorry. What was the question? I must have missed it.

Absence Epilepsy

Absence epilepsy is a common form of generalized epilepsy seen in children. Typical seizures are characterized by sudden episodes of loss of responsiveness with staring and behavioral arrest lasting for 10–30 seconds. Such seizures are referred to as dialeptic seizures.

During these episodes, patients may also have automatisms such as rhythmic head-nodding, lip-smacking, and/or blinking. After each episode, the child returns completely back to normal, showing no signs of a postictal state. The seizures can be subtle and can be overlooked for sometime, often being misdiagnosed as inattention.

The EEG hallmark of absence epilepsy is a generalized burst of spike and slow wave discharges, lasting for at least 3 seconds, known as 3 Hz spike and wave. These discharges are often provoked with hyperventilation.

The standard treatment is ethosuximide, which blocks T-type Ca^{2+} channels. Some patients could also have generalized tonic–clonic (GTC) seizures, in addition to dialeptic seizures. Ethosuximide is not an effective treatment for GTC seizures, and such patients often require an additional anti-seizure medication, such as levetiracetam or lamotrigine.

The prognosis of childhood absence epilepsy is very good with high rates of remission. On the other hand, juvenile absence epilepsy has a variable course and the remission rates are lower.

17

• • • • •

First the ankle, then toward peak,
Spreading numb but mostly weak,
No reflex, or cells of white,
But proteins high, not from tick bite.

Hint #1

First the flu, and now this?

Hint #2

If you missed it, drop the F-wave.

Acute Inflammatory Demyelinating Polyradiculoneuropathy

The most common form of Guillain–Barre syndrome (GBS), acute inflammatory demyelinating polyradiculoneurolopathy (AIDP) is an immune-mediated disorder that targets the peripheral nerves and accounts for up to 90% of all cases of GBS. Patients with AIDP present with subacute symmetrical progressive weakness and paresthesias, along with significantly decreased or absent tendon reflexes. Though patients commonly complain of an ascending pattern of lower extremity weakness and sensory changes, this is not always the case. In over half of these patients, neurological symptoms are preceded by a nonspecific febrile illness, or gastrointestinal or respiratory infections days to weeks prior to symptom onset. The most common preceding infectious cause is *Campylobacter jejuni* gastroenteritis. However, many other antecedent infections have been associated with the later development of AIDP, including Epstein–Barr virus, hepatitis virus, *Mycoplasma* pneumonia, cytomegalovirus, and HIV. Additionally, metabolically stressful events have been known to precede the onset of AIDP symptoms, such as pregnancy, surgery, extreme emotional and physical stress, vaccination, and development of another autoimmune disease.

Symptoms in the majority of patients begin with a vague paresthesias and/or a feeling of "numbness" in the feet and hands. This progression does not follow a length-dependent (glove and stocking) pattern. A few days after the onset of sensory changes, the patients often report experiencing weakness that follows the same symmetrical ascending pattern. Weakness is often profound and can result in complete paralysis of the affected limbs, reaching its peak effect between two and four weeks. Additionally, in approximately half of patients with AIDP, facial weakness and cranial nerve involvement is seen. The involvement of the respiratory muscles can be life-threatening, and the patient may require mechanical ventilation. Further complicating the care of those with AIDP is the autonomic instability. These patients experience large fluctuations in both heart rate and blood pressure as well as a predisposition to the development of cardiac arrhythmias.

Diagnosis of AIDP is clinical. Supporting evidence is often acquired via a lumbar puncture. The most characteristic CSF abnormality is albumino-cytologic dissociation, which is a high protein level with normal cell count. This finding is present in ~50–66% of cases in week 1 and > 75% of cases in week 3.

Electromyography is also most sensitive if performed several weeks after the onset of symptoms, with nerve conduction studies showing peripheral nerve demyelination as well as the absence of F-waves in the early stages of AIDP.

Treatment of AIDP usually includes either plasmapheresis or IV immunoglobulin. The choice depends upon feasibility, availability, and patient preference. The prognosis of AIDP is generally good, with the majority of patients returning to their normal baseline function after acute treatment and subsequent rehabilitation; however AIDP is fatal in 5% of cases.

18

• • • • •

Several hours, pulsing pains,
Dim lit room after it rains,
Some have signs at times before,
Abort by shrinking vessel bore.

Migraine Headache

Migraine headache is experienced by approximately 18% of women and 6% of men. It is the most common cause of headache-related medical visits.

The pathophysiology of migraine consists of a phenomenon called cortical spreading depression of Leão. This is a traveling wave of depolarization that spreads across the cerebral cortex and is directly related to the various manifestations of migraine. This phenomenon is responsible for the various auras experienced by migraine patients. The cortical spreading depression also activates the trigeminal afferent nerve fibers. These afferent fibers originate from the pseudounipolar neurons in the trigeminal ganglion and they project to the small and large cranial blood vessels. Activation of this trigeminal system leads to the release of vasoactive peptides like CGRP (calcitonin gene-related peptide), substance P, and neurokinin A. This leads to a sterile neurogenic inflammation associated with vasodilation. Peripheral and central sensitization of the neurons leads to intensification of the pain, and decreased pain threshold, and makes the neurons very responsive to both nociceptive and non-nociceptive stimuli.

Symptoms of migraine can vary significantly based on if the patient is having a "typical migraine" or one of the many migraine variants such as basilar migraine, hemiplegic migraine, vestibular migraine, and acephalgic migraine. Patients with a typical migraine often complain of attacks of unilateral or bilateral moderate to severe intensity head pain that have a pulsatile quality, last hours to days, and are aggravated by physical activity. During migraine attacks there is often associate nausea, vomiting, and sensitivity to light and sound. Though approximately 80% of patients with migraine do not experience a preceding aura, those that do often report experiencing one or more visual (flickering light and/or blind spots), sensory (paresthesias and/or numbness), or vocal (dysphasic) symptoms minutes to hours prior to migraine-type pain.

The treatment of migraine headaches consists of abortive and preventive therapy. Abortive medications include NSAIDs, triptans, steroids, antiemetics, ergot derivatives, and CGRP antagonists. Currently, rimegepant and ubrogepant have positive clinical trials supporting their use as abortive therapy. Preventive therapy includes medications like propranolol, anticonvulsants (topiramate, valproate), verapamil, tricyclic antidepressants, and CGRP antagonists. The CGRP antagonists have revolutionized migraine treatment. Currently available options include erenumab, fremanezumab, and galcanezumab. Most of these are administered via subcutaneous or intravenous routes. Botulinum toxin injections are also approved for preventive therapy.

19

• • • • •

Uncommon mimicker in those,
With shaking and shuffling toes,
But eyes cannot look up or downward,
You'll sometimes see a hummingbird.

Hint #1

The answer is tangled and tufted.

Hint #2

You will not hallucinate the correct answer.

Progressive Supranuclear Palsy

Progressive supranuclear palsy (PSP) (Steele–Richardson–Olszewski syndrome) is a neurodegenerative disease, which presents with atypical Parkinsonism or a Parkinson-plus syndrome. PSP is a tauopathy, characterized by the formation of tau-positive neurofibrillary tangles, tufted astrocytes, and glial loss, all primarily in the brainstem nuclei, basal ganglia, and frontal lobes.

Clinical signs and symptoms are similar to Parkinson disease (PD). Like PD, individuals exhibit axial rigidity, cognitive impairment, postural instability, and gait freezing with frequent falls; however, gait is often more wide-based than shuffling. The development of freezing gait and unprovoked falls within the first few years of symptom onset is more specific for PSP. Abnormal eye movements can help provide a key differentiation from PD, as patients with PSP often experience supranuclear gaze palsy, especially vertical gaze palsy, ocular square wave jerks, and slow saccades. A very early subtle exam finding before obvious vertical gaze limitation is slowing of catch-up saccades with vertical OKN (optokinetic nystagmus). The impaired gaze seen in PSP often starts with impaired voluntary downward gaze, then progresses to impaired voluntary upward gaze and then lateral gaze.

Cognitive impairment is seen in >50% of patients with PSP and develops early within the first few years of disease onset. Cognitive testing in these patients often shows impaired executive function parameters such as planning, complex task performance, and reasoning.

Imaging in these patients is often normal; however, a minority of cases will show noticeable dorsal, rostral and caudal midbrain tegmentum atrophy on brain MRI, which when seen on midsagittal view resembles a hummingbird (hummingbird sign). The use of more advanced imaging techniques, such as Tau-positron emission tomography (PET) and DaT scan, shows limited sensitivity and specificity, however, these are still being studied for their use in diagnosing PSP.

Prognosis is very poor in patients with PSP, and life expectancy after symptoms onset is much shorter than that of PD, with median life-expectancy being 5–6 years. Unfortunately, there are no good treatment options and management mostly relies on support and prevention of falls.

20

• • • • •

Eyelid weakness, vision double,
If no treatment, breathing trouble,
Postsynaptic 'ceptors bare,
Replace the humor, treat the flare.

Hint #1

The correct answer might also be tough to swallow.

Hint #2

The answer may be a block by an antibody.

Myasthenia Gravis

Myasthenia gravis (MG) is an acquired antibody-mediated auto-immune disease of the neuromuscular junction. The pathophysiology is widely studied and overall well understood. In MG, the binding of antibodies with nicotinic acetylcholine receptor (AChR) and other proteins (e.g., muscle-specific kinase, MuSK) to the postsynaptic membrane result in decreased binding of Ach to the receptors and increased destruction of the receptors. There are several other antibodies found in patients with MG such as lipoprotein-related protein 4 antibodies (LRP4), titin antibodies, ryanodine receptor antibodies (RyR), and voltage-gated potassium channel antibodies (VGKC); however, their prevalence is relatively low and their sensitivity and specificity to MG is still under study. Thymic lymphofolliculuar hyperplasia is common in patients with MG (70%); however, thymic tumor (thymoma) is only seen in 10% of patients. Symptoms present more commonly in women in their 20s and 30s and in men in their 50s and 60s, with overall higher prevalence in women.

Symptoms of MG most commonly include fatigable oculobulbar and proximal muscle weakness presenting as ptosis, diplopia, dysphagia, dysarthria, as well as jaw, neck, proximal limb (arms > legs), truck, and respiratory muscle weakness. Ocular symptoms are often bilateral but asymmetric. Ocular symptoms are most common in MG, with some patients with MG having symptoms isolated to only ptosis and diplopia (ocular MG). Symptoms of MG characteristically get worse throughout the day and with repeated use, and improve with rest. These symptoms can become life-threatening in approximately 20% of patients. Severe exacerbations can result in *myasthenic crisis*, which can be life-threatening because of severe impairment of respiratory and bulbar function, requiring intubation and mechanical ventilation. Myasthenic crises are often precipitated by a physical or metabolic insult such as surgery or infection.

Both sensitive and specific clinical signs of MG can be easily elicited on physical exam. These tests typically exploit the inherent fatigability of the muscles by asking the patient to perform isometric or dynamic exercises to look for the proceeding muscle fatigue. This can be done by using sustained upgaze to find subsequent ptosis and diplopia and sustained arm abduction to find subsequent shoulder weakness, among other tests.

Bloodwork to establish a diagnosis should include AChR-binding antibodies, AChR-modulating antibodies, and AChR-blocking antibodies, with AChR-binding antibodies being the most sensitive. If these are negative, 40% of patients with underlying MG will be MuSK antibody positive. If AChR and MuSK antibodies are negative but clinical suspicion remains high, LRP4 antibodies may be positive in approximately 7% of otherwise seronegative patients.

Though routine EMG and nerve conduction studies are often normal in MG, slow repetitive nerve stimulation can show a decrement in CMAP amplitude. The most sensitive diagnostic test for MG is single-fiber electromyography. This relies on the principle of detecting variability of action potential latencies between two muscle fibers, innervated by the same motor unit. This variability is called "jitter."

The treatment mainly relies on symptomatic management with pyridostigmine and disease modification with immunotherapies. Steroids are often the first choice. Other agents like azathioprine or mycophenolate are also started with steroids, and once they have had enough time to work, steroids are tapered off. Newer therapies such as efgartigimod alfa and ravulizumab are also available now. Thymectomy must be done in patients with thymoma. If thymoma is not present but the patient has generalized MG and is at an age ≤ 50 years, thymectomy must be offered.

21

• • • • •

Sudden symptoms head pain and,
LP will show red cells, no band,
CT with white is sensitive,
Secure then channel blockers give.

Hint #1

The answer will hit you like a thunderclap.

Hint #2

If you do not know, ask either Hunt, Hess, or Fisher.

Subarachnoid Hemorrhage

Representing 5–10% of all strokes, idiopathic subarachnoid hemorrhages are most commonly caused by ruptured intracranial saccular aneurysms (~80%), with the remainder caused by vascular malformations and ruptured mycotic/infective aneurysms. Subarachnoid hemorrhage can also be seen with co-occurring intracerebral hemorrhage and trauma.

Patients with subarachnoid hemorrhage often present to the hospital with either acute onset "worst headache of life," aka "thunderclap headache," vomiting, neck pain, seizures, or abrupt alterations in consciousness. Additionally, some patients can identify a severe but brief headache episode, preceding the hospitalization by many days or weeks. This first severe headache is often considered the "sentinel hemorrhage," which is thought to be a small bleed that occurs at the aneurysm site prior to the major aneurysm rupture.

Easily and often first seen on non-contrasted CT imaging, subarachnoid hemorrhage appears as hyperdensity commonly seen in the basal cisterns, sylvian fissures, and interhemispheric cisterns, as well as at the base of the brain surrounding the circle of Willis. These non-contrasted studies may also show hyperdense blood products inside the ventricles and co-occurring ventricular dilation representing intraventricular hemorrhage and hydrocephalus, respectively. The most common location of intracranial aneurysms is in the anterior circulation, for example, anterior communicating artery, posterior communicating artery, and bifurcation of the middle cerebral artery. The severity of subarachnoid hemorrhage is graded in terms of symptom severity using the Hunt–Hess grading scale, and the extent of subarachnoid and intraventricular blood using the modified Fisher grading scale.

If non-contrasted CT is suggestive of subarachnoid hemorrhage, CT angiography is often the next imaging of choice, and if negative despite high clinical suspicion for a ruptured aneurysm, the gold standard imaging modality is digital subtraction angiography. A lumbar puncture is also indicated if the suspicion is considerable and imaging inconclusive, with a positive LP showing pigmented hemoglobin breakdown products (xanthochromia).

Some of the most significant complications of subarachnoid hemorrhage include obstructive hydrocephalus and elevated intracranial pressure, delayed cerebral ischemia due to cerebral vasospasm, seizures, hyponatremia, and Takotsubo cardiomyopathy.

Patients with subarachnoid hemorrhage must be managed in an ICU, preferably a neurosurgical ICU. Treatment includes early identification of the culprit aneurysm and securing it with either embolization or clipping. Obstructive hydrocephalus requires placement of an external ventriculostomy catheter. The current accepted standard of care for prevention of cerebral vasospasm is to use nimodipine, a calcium channel blocker, and to maintain euvolemia in all patients with aneurysmal subarachnoid hemorrhage. If and when clinical cerebral vasospasm does develop, the patient must be aggressively treated with pressor agents like phenylephrine or norepinephrine. Intra-arterial vasodilators like verapamil, papaverine, or milrinone may also be required for more refractory cases.

22

• • • • •

Both spastic and fasciculations,
In three regions of these patients,
EMG will fibrillate,
Block presynaptic glutamate.

Amyotrophic Lateral Sclerosis

First termed by Jean-Martin Charcot in 1874, amyotrophic lateral sclerosis (ALS), also known as Lou Gehrig's disease, is the most common motor neuron disease in adults, affecting approximately 1 person per 100,000 people per year. Most cases of ALS arise as a sporadic neurodegenerative disease, though approximately 5% of cases are inherited. Of the inherited forms of ALS, the most common genetic mutation affects the C9orf72 gene. Mutations of genes such as SOD1 (superoxide dismutase 1) and FUS (*fused in sarcoma*) have been implicated in the development of inherited juvenile ALS.

Clinical findings of ALS include upper motor neuron (UMN) signs such as spasticity, increased tendon reflexes, and Babinski sign, co-occurring with lower motor neuron (LMN) signs such as muscle fasciculations, muscle wasting, and hyporeflexia. The totality of these exam findings allows the provider to group rate the likelihood that the patient has ALS by setting criteria for suspected, possible, clinically probable, probable, and definite ALS. For example, if the patient has UMN and LMN in only one leg, the patient meets criteria for "possible ALS," while UMN and LMN signs in ≥ 3 body regions is considered "definite ALS." It is also imperative to assess cognitive symptoms. It is well known that frontotemporal dementia (FTD) and motor neuron disease (MND) form a spectrum. This is especially true in inherited forms of ALS as with C9orf72 mutation.

Since ALS is almost always a fatal diagnosis, it is absolutely necessary to rule out potential mimickers, for example, cervical myelopathy (predominant UMN signs in all extremities), multifocal motor neuropathy with conduction block, inflammatory myopathies, and so on. NCS/EMG often plays a critical role in excluding alternative diagnoses.

Though ALS is a 100% fatal neurodegenerative disease, medications such as riluzole and edaravone are available and have been shown to prolong life-expectancy by months. Due to the progressive dysphagia and respiratory muscle weakness, patients with ALS will eventually require alternative means of nutrition and ventilation to survive. Most patients with ALS live 3–5 years after symptom onset. Recently, media attention has been paid to ALS after the very popular 2014 ice bucket challenge was developed to raise money for ALS research.

23

• • • • •

Mid frequency and amplitude,
And no effect on eyes or mood,
Alcohol provides an aid,
And treatment with beta blockade.

Hint #1

You will not find the answer at rest.

Hint #2

The answer on the most common of its kind.

Essential Tremor

Essential tremor is a progressive, chronic action tremor that is most commonly found in the bilateral hands and arms (90%); however, it can also be found in the head and neck (30%), legs (12%), and voice (20%). Though symptoms can be disabling for some, in most cases symptoms are only mild and do not require medical intervention. There also appears to be a large proportion of patients (50%–70%) who show an autosomal dominant familial transmission.

The tremor of ET is approx. 4–10 Hz, mostly symmetrical, evident with action, and absent at rest. Both posture against gravity and voluntary movement make the tremor evident or worse, and often patients report difficulty with writing, eating with utensils, and drinking from a glass. Approximately half of those with ET can experience a transient improvement in their symptoms with alcohol ingestion. In addition to the predominant tremor features, up to half of these patients also exhibit signs of cerebellar dysfunction such as gait ataxia. Key differentiators from Parkinson disease are the absence of tremor at rest, the absence of limb rigidity, the absence of face or tongue tremor, and that it is not uncommonly found in patients in their 20s and 30s.

The diagnosis is clinical. The first-line treatment for essential tremor is propranolol. If there are significant contraindications or no benefit, another treatment option is primidone. Propranolol and primidone can be used in a combination. Second-line treatment options include gabapentin, topiramate, and benzodiazepines. In refractory cases, deep brain stimulation (DBS) therapy targeted at the Vim (Ventral intermediate) nucleus of the thalamus or stereotactic thalamotomy can be offered.

24

• • • • •

High CK and EMG,
Show spontaneous activity,
Weakness, pain and Anti-Jo,
No rash but should biopsy though.

Hint #1

After finding the answer, give steroids.

Hint #2

Associated with autoimmune conditions.

Polymyositis

Polymyositis is an autoimmune condition (thought to be T-cell mediated) resulting in muscle inflammation and destruction that can occur as an isolated syndrome or as a part of any of several systemic autoimmune diseases such as Crohn disease, systemic lupus, celiac disease, Sjogren syndrome, Behcet's, sarcoidosis, and many others. Polymyositis can be differentiated from dermatomyositis by findings on muscle biopsy and the absence of dermatological findings.

Patients with polymyositis often exhibit a characteristic progressive, symmetric, proximal muscle weakness that develops over the course of weeks and can be preceded by infections, commonly in the upper respiratory tract. Like patients with dermatomyositis, patients with polymyositis report significant muscle pain and tenderness and significant weakness in their hips and shoulders. Additionally, cardiac involvement occurs in approximately 40% of patients with polymyositis and can result in arrhythmias, myocarditis, conduction defects, and congestive heart failure. Pulmonary manifestations are particularly common in a subtype of polymyositis called antisynthetase syndrome.

Bloodwork often shows an elevated CK ~50x greater than normal; however, patients can have normal levels, even with active disease. Other muscle enzymes such as lactate dehydrogenase, aldolase, and aminotransferase may also be elevated in polymyositis. Antibodies such as anti-Jo-1 (aminoacyl-tRNA synthetase) are common in the antisynthetase subtype.

On electromyography, inflammation and myonecrosis can be indicated by diffuse spontaneous activity (fibrillation potentials and positive sharp waves). In addition, myopathic motor units are also seen. Muscle biopsy shows necrotic muscle fibers, inflammatory endomysial infiltration, and muscle atrophy.

Treatment includes steroids and steroid sparing agents like azathioprine and methotrexate.

25

· · · · ·

Abnormal movements and mentation,
Trinuclear anticipation,
In younger and in family,
On chromosome 4, and gene HTT.

Hint #1

The answer is as easy as C,A,G-1,2,3.

Hint #2

As you think, the caudates shrink (and putamen).

Huntington Disease

Huntington disease (HD) is an autosomal dominant neurodegenerative disease resulting from the trinucleotide repeat expansion of (CAG) sequence on chromosome 4, HTT gene, in exon 1. These CAG trinucleotide repeats (<35 repeats) are seen in individuals without HD, though all individuals with ≥40 CAG repeats develop HD, and those with ≥60 often develop juvenile HD. The average age of onset is 35–45 years.

The clinical hallmark of HD is obviously chorea. These movements are quick, random, and purposeless and have a flowing but unpredictable pattern. The distribution of chorea in HD can be quite diffuse and variable, but special attention must be paid to the forehead. Choreiform movements affecting the forehead are extremely unlikely to occur in any condition other than HD. These patients also develop dystonia, motor impersistence, eye movement abnormalities, and significant behavioral and cognitive impairment.

Motor impersistence is often tested by asking the patient to stick out their tongue and to hold it in that position. Patients often have difficulty doing this for more than 5 seconds and the tongue moves in and out (fly-catcher's tongue). It can also be tested in extremities by asking the patient to squeeze the examiner's fingers. The examiner can feel the impersistence of this movement, referred to as milkmaid's grip.

One of the earliest motor signs in HD patients before unequivocal chorea develops is oculomotor apraxia. Patients use head thrusts to direct voluntary saccades.

Though MRI is not required for definitive diagnosis, atrophy of the caudate and putamen is often evident, along with significant dilation of the lateral ventricles. Genetic testing must be performed in all individuals suspected of having HD or with a strong family history of HD.

HD is a fatal disease. For symptomatic management of chorea, VMAT-2 inhibitors like tetrabenazine and deutetrabenazine are used. If there is severe comorbid depression or psychosis, atypical antipsychotics can be used instead of, for example, olanzapine, risperidone, or aripiprazole. Patients on VMAT-2 inhibitors must be closely monitored for worsening depression or suicidal ideation.

26

• • • • •

Rapid dement, mood liability,
On MRI, bright glowing you'll see,
Pulvinar sign, and with a back prick,
14 double 3, positive RT Quic.

Hint #1

Look no further than the humble hockey stick.

Hint #2

Think diffuse vacuolization.

79

Creutzfeldt–Jakob Disease

Occurring in approximately 1 per 1,000,000 people yearly worldwide, Creutzfeldt–Jakob disease (CJD) is the most common form of prion disease. Prion diseases are a group of neurodegenerative disorders that results from the abnormal accumulation of a cell surface glycoprotein called prion protein (PrP), which is encoded by the prion gene PRNP on chromosome 20. Interestingly, PrP is normally found in healthy brains; however, for an unknown reason, and by an unknown mechanism, normal PrP undergoes a posttranslational conformational change that makes it insoluble and resistant to protease degradation. These abnormal forms of PrP then self-propagate and convert normal forms of PrP to pathological forms like themselves. Though there are no known environmental or modifiable risk factors currently known for CJD, there is a genetic risk factor, which is homozygosity of the codon 129 on PRNP gene. Although 90% of CJD is sporadic, there are also familial and iatrogenic forms.

Typical clinical presentation is a rapidly progressive dementia with myoclonus. The cognitive and behavioral changes seen in CJD are often the most significant and commonly include aphasias, memory and concentration impairment, hallucinations, and delusions. Additionally, focal weakness and ataxia are not uncommon. In the later stages, startle myoclonus can be seen in ~80% of patients. Prior to death, which is often only 4–6 months after symptom onset, these patients eventually deteriorate to a state of akinetic-mutism.

CSF analysis often shows normal or mildly elevated protein in the setting of normal cell count and glucose. Other nonspecific markers of neuronal damage such as neuron-specific enolase, 14–3-3, and S100 protein may be elevated but are not sensitive or specific to CJD. The most sensitive and specific CSF analysis currently available is the real-time quaking-induced conversion assay, also known as RT-QuIC.

EEG can also be used to help diagnose CJD in the right clinical context and often shows generalized background slowing in the early disease stages but develops into synchronous periodic sharp wave complexes (biphasic and/or triphasic) in the mid-late stages, and returning back to generalized background slowing as the patient approaches the end stages of CJD.

MRI can also be very useful in confirming the diagnosis of CJD, with increased signal seen on DWI and FLAIR sequences in the striatum as well as cortical ribboning in two or more lobes. Additionally, bilateral FLAIR hyperintensity can be seen in bilateral dorsal thalami, known as the pulvinar sign or hockey stick sign. The most definitive test that can be performed to diagnose CJD is brain biopsy. Histopathology shows spongiform changes with neuronal loss, astrocytic gliosis, and neuropil vacuolation.

27

• • • • •

In compromised, Low CD4,
From uncooked meat, poop picked off floor,
Multiple ring-enhanced are seen,
Treat with pyrimethamine.

CNS Toxoplasmosis

An opportunistic infection occurring in severely immunocompromised individuals, for example, those with AIDS, toxoplasmosis of the central nervous system most often occurs when the patients' CD4 T-lymphocyte count falls below 200. Toxoplasma gondii is acquired by ingesting contaminated water, food (uncooked meat), or by handling cat feces.

Most patients with CNS toxoplasmosis will present with subacute signs and symptoms of fever, headache, altered mental status, and focal neurological deficits, though approximately 25% of patients with CNS toxoplasmosis will present with seizure. In rare cases, patients with CNS toxoplasmosis have presented with encephalitis, spinal cord toxoplasmosis, hemiballismus, and hemichorea.

MRI of the brain usually shows multiple, space-occupying, ring-enhancing lesions that have surrounding vasogenic edema, most commonly found in the gray–white junction and basal ganglia. Bloodwork testing for serum toxoplasmosis IgG antibody titer can help indicate previous exposure; however, these results alone are not sufficient to diagnose or rule out CNS toxoplasmosis as an immunocompromised state can blunt the antibody response, yielding unreliable results. Performing a lumbar puncture is often considered high risk in these patients with known brain lesions, and CSF analysis is often unhelpful unless clinical suspicion is high, as CSF toxoplasmosis DNA polymerase chain reaction (PCR) analysis often lacks sensitivity.

Differential diagnoses include any other opportunistic infection and CNS lymphoma. An AIDS patient with multiple ring-enhancing lesions on MRI and a positive toxoplasma IgG must be empirically treated with sulfadiazine and pyrimethamine. Atovaquone can also be used.

28

• • • • •

Often spotted at young age,
Averted eyes, does not engage,
Interests few, of those intense,
Broad *spectrum* of intelligence.

Hint #1

General scientific consensus is that the condition has nothing to do
with vaccination.

Hint #2

Hold onto the answer, much like individuals with this disorder hold onto echolalia.

Autism Spectrum Disorder

Autism spectrum disorder (ASD) is a neurodevelopmental disorder characterized by impairment of social communication skills and repetitive behaviors.

The diagnosis is usually made before two years of age. Early signs and symptoms include impaired or delayed language and social skills, avoidance of eye contact, and obsessive and repetitive behaviors. The DMS-5 criteria require all these features to be present for the diagnosis along with impaired functioning.

Routine bloodwork and imaging in these individuals is often normal. The gold standard for diagnosis is the autism diagnostic observational scale (ADOS), which requires multiple hours and certified examiners. Supplementary testing is available and can be administered by a caregiver at home, including the autism diagnostic index-revised (ADI-R). Referral to genetics or genetic evaluation by chromosomal microarray is increasingly becoming the standard of care.

Treatment of children with ASD often requires a multidisciplinary approach, especially if ASD exists with other medical comorbidities like epilepsy. Early diagnosis and intervention are critical for improved functioning. Multiple providers including neurologists, psychologists, geneticists, occupational therapists, speech therapists, and social workers are required for effective treatment. These children must be placed in a special-education program in the school. The Individuals with Disabilities Education Act in the United States assures that such education is provided for free in public schools.

29

• • • • •

Double vision, eyelids low,
Trouble with chewing and swallow,
Weakness downward in those who,
Eat from honey/home-canned food.

Hint #1

Weakness starts from the top.

Hint #2

You know the answer. What are you waiting spore?

Botulism

Caused by *Clostridium botulinum* – a neurotoxic, spore-forming, obligate anaerobic bacilli – botulism is most commonly acquired by ingesting the toxin through home-canned or home-processed foods, or ingesting the preformed spores by infants. Botulism can also be acquired through a wound, as *C botulinum* is commonly found in the soil.

Once the toxin is absorbed into the bloodstream, it irreversibly binds and is internalized by presynaptic nerve endings of both cranial nerves and peripheral nerves. The toxin then cleaves essential polypeptides needed for the docking and eventual release of acetylcholine from the presynaptic membrane.

Symptoms of botulism develop over time; however, in the food-borne form of botulism, symptoms begin within the first 36 hours and consist of diarrhea, nausea, and vomiting, though constipation is often a later symptom. In wound botulism there are no gastro-intestinal symptoms. A few days after ingestion, the first neuro-logical signs of botulism usually include oculobulbar symptoms such as diplopia, dysphagia, dry mouth, dysphonia, and blurry vision (due to fixed and dilated pupils). Weakness continues in a downward progression and from proximal to distal, starting with the cranial nerves, then affecting the neck, upper extremities, trunk, and then lower extremities. Respiratory weakness is common and can be severe, requiring intubation and mechanical ventilation. Autonomic involvement is common, and these patients also suffer from constipation, urinary retention, and orthostatic hypotension. On exam, in addition to weakness, patients will often have absent tendon reflexes and unreactive pupils.

The diagnosis can be made by detecting botulinum toxin in the serum or stool or *C botulinum* bacteria in the stool.

In addition to providing standard supportive and intensive care to patients, the main treatment option is the antitoxin. The state health department must immediately be informed of a suspected botulism case and to acquire the antitoxin from the CDC.

30

• • • • •

One-way eyes, other sided weak,
And on CT darkness you seek,
Arm shows drift, but leg may not,
Ignore left, if this side clots.

Large Right Middle Cerebral Artery Territory Cerebral Infarct

Cerebral strokes are the leading cause of severe neurological disability in adults, with approximately 75% of strokes being ischemic in nature, causing cerebral infarction. They are caused by a localized reduction in sufficient blood flow that results in the disruption of normal neuronal metabolism and function. Generally speaking, approximately 30% of all ischemic strokes are caused by a cardioembolism, ~20% from large artery atherosclerotic disease, ~20% are small subcortical "lacunar" infarcts, and ~30% have undetermined cause and are labeled cryptogenic.

The symptoms of large right middle cerebral artery (MCA) territory cerebral infarcts vary widely depending on how distal the arterial obstruction lies and the amount of collateral blood flow the patient had from adjacent arterial territories. In general, large right MCA territory infarcts will cause ischemia to the majority of right frontal and parietal lobes, and a significant portion of the temporal lobe, without ischemia to the occipital lobe or cerebellum. Typical symptoms include left arm and leg weakness (arm is usually worse than leg), a left homonymous hemianopia, and neglect of the left hemi-environment. Because language dominance is usually in the left hemisphere, it is most often preserved in large right hemispheric MCA infarctions. Patients may however display dysarthria.

The left hemi-spatial neglect can be quite subtle where the patient does acknowledge the existence of the left side of the world, but neglect can be detected by giving simultaneous stimuli in both fields and asking the patient to detect them. The patient usually ignores the one in the left hemifield. This is called extinction. In more severe forms, patients ignore the left side of their environment. Sometimes, they are unaware of their own left-sided weakness, known as anosognosia. In extreme cases, they also deny the existence of their left body and ascribe them to the examiner, a condition known as somatoparaphrenia.

Subacute cerebral infarcts appear as hypodense on non-contrast CT; however, infarcts occurring <3 hours since symptom onset often appear isodense with the adjacent healthy tissue. The Alberta Stroke Program Early CT Scoring (ASPECTS) test is a recently developed standardized scoring system that measures the distribution of hypodensity found on non-contrasted CT and can help estimate the infarct size and risk of hemorrhagic conversion, and helps screen for possible further intervention with mechanical thrombectomy.

31

• • • • •

Memory, language, judgment, praxis,
Prior to five on the third axis,
Plaques throughout and tangles in,
Those with mutated PSEN.

Hint #1

Line 2 references the DSM-IV.

Hint #2

More common in Down Syndrome than neuro-typical individuals.

Alzheimer Disease

Alzheimer disease (AD) is the most common form of dementia in the elderly and is seen in ~15% of people of 75 years and ~30% of those above 85 years old. Although the exact cause of AD is unknown, the histopathology is relatively well understood as the accumulation of extracellular β–amyloid plaques and intracellular neurofibrillary tangles made of abnormally phosphorylated tau protein.

Most cases of AD are thought to be sporadic, though there are specific genes that are passed by autosomal dominant inheritance. The genes presenilin-1 and presenilin-2, and amyloid precursor protein (PSEN 1, PSEN 2, and APP) are inherited via autosomal dominant pattern, and if inherited they bring an almost 100% chance of developing early-onset AD, with symptoms usually beginning prior to the age of 60. The APOE (apolipoprotein E) gene is mainly implicated in late-onset AD. The ε4 allele of APOE gene in particular confers a risk of developing late-onset AD. Genetic testing and genetic counseling is recommended in families with early-onset dementia.

The earliest and most prominent features of AD are short-term memory loss, impaired judgment, and deficits in executive function and visuospatial navigation. It is thought that there is a considerable number of years of amyloid plaque and tangle deposition prior to symptom onset. Initially, cognitive impairment is noticed on cognitive screening assessments such as the mini mental state exam (MMSE) or the Montreal cognitive assessment (MoCA). There are no routine blood tests that can be performed to diagnose AD though reversible causes of cognitive decline should be ruled out (vitamin deficiency, metabolic disease, infection). Likewise, lumbar puncture can be a helpful way to rule out mimicking infectious, inflammatory, and neoplastic CNS causes.

Additional CSF analysis of β-amyloid-42 and tau currently have unknown utility; however, it may be useful in early-onset AD.

As with any individual with dementia, imaging with CT or MRI is indicated. Best seen on MRI, patients with moderate to advanced stage AD show bilateral hippocampal and parietal atrophy. Interestingly, prior to the publication of the fourth version of the Diagnostic and Statistical Manual (DSM-4), AD was listed as an "axis 3" mental illness; however, this designation was not continued into the DSM-5 version.

Until most recently, the treatment of AD was mostly symptomatic with modest benefit at best. Cholinesterase inhibitors (donepezil, rivastigmine, and galantamine) are usually indicated in anyone with a new diagnosis of AD. For more severe cases, memantine (NMDA-receptor antagonist) is recommended. The US FDA approved aducanumab (a recombinant monoclonal antibody against amyloid beta) for the treatment of AD in 2021, but its use is still considered controversial and many experts do not agree that it offers significant benefit for its cost.

32

• • • • •

Most common of benign subset,
And more commonly in women yet,
They push from outward in, grow slow,
Often get big, you may not know.

Hint #1

The answer is well-defined.

Hint #2

Do not give up, no matter what.

Meningioma

Representing ~35% of all primary brain tumors, meningiomas are also the most common benign brain tumors. Meningiomas most commonly present in the third and fourth decade of life and are 3 times more common in women than in men. Approximately 90% of meningiomas arise supratentorially, growing from the dural arachnoidal cap cells. Though they very rarely invade brain tissue, they often grow slowly, can get very large before causing neurological symptoms, and are commonly found incidentally on brain imaging. The most common known risk factor is exposure to ionizing radiation. Radiation-induced meningiomas are more likely to have cellular atypia. As far as genetic risk factors are concerned, the most significant is perhaps neurofibromatosis 2 (NF2). About half of NF2 patients have meningiomas and usually they have multiple meningiomas.

Initial presenting symptoms of meningioma range widely, but patients most commonly complain of headache syndromes, progressive focal weakness, or seizures. Meningiomas are typically easily identifiable as a well-defined mass with smooth or lobulated consistency, appearing isodense or hyperdense on non-contrasted CT. On MRI, this extra-axial tumor is usually isointense or hypointense on T1 and isointense or hyperintense on T2/FLAIR, but it shows very homogenous enhancement on T1 post-gadolinium sequence with a "dural tail."

The treatment of choice for large or symptomatic meningiomas is surgical resection. The WHO Grade I meningiomas, when resected completely, do not require any additional therapy. WHO Grade III meningiomas require radiation therapy in addition to surgical resection to decrease the risk of recurrence.

33

• • • • •

Febrile seizure on one side,
But afterward they do not reside,
Crouch'ed gait with outward feet,
And highly sensitive to heat.

Hint #1

Onset within the first year of life.

Hint #2

Eventual developmental delay.

Dravet Syndrome

Dravet syndrome is a type of developmental epileptic encephalopathy (DEE), which typically begins in the first year of life with a febrile hemi-clonic seizure. This later progresses to more frequent, prolonged afebrile seizure types including focal and generalized clonic, myoclonic, and atypical absence seizures that are refractory to treatment. Within a year of seizure onset, developmental delay becomes evident and the child eventually shows profound cognitive and behavioral deficits. Because of frequent convulsive seizures, the patients with Dravet syndrome have a much higher risk of sudden unexpected death in epilepsy (SUDEP) at ~9.3 per 1000 patient-years, which is almost the same as adults with drug-resistant epilepsy. In fact, the most common cause of death in Dravet syndrome is SUDEP.

In the majority of cases, Dravet syndrome is caused by a loss-of-function mutation in the SCN1A gene, which codes for a voltage-gated Na^+ channel, mainly located on the inhibitory interneurons.

Interestingly, despite often normal timing and quality of gait formation, by adolescence, patients with Dravet syndrome develop a characteristic crouched gait. Also, somewhat unique to individuals with Dravet syndrome is the heightened sensitivity to changes in bodily and environmental temperature, as seizures can often be triggered by hot baths, low-grade fevers, physical exercise, and even warm ambient air.

In about half of the patients, the EEG demonstrates abnormal slowing of the background rhythm whereas the other half could have a normal background rhythm up to five years of age. The interictal epileptiform discharges are usually generalized or multifocal.

Anti-seizure medications form the cornerstone of management. Typically, the first-line treatment includes valproate and clobazam.

The second-line options include topiramate, stiripentol, fenfluramine, and cannabidiol. Fenfluramine is the most recently approved treatment for Dravet syndrome. In the pivotal trials published, none of the patients developed valvular abnormalities or pulmonary hypertension.

34

• • • • •

Cannot look right when flow gets light,
And on CT, the brain's not bright,
The right side will be strength seeking,
And patients have trouble speaking.

Hint #1

Often rank highly on the NIH stroke scale.

Hint #2

Exam more likely to be atypical if left-handed.

Large Left Middle Cerebral Artery Territory Infarct

The left hemisphere is usually considered the "dominant" hemisphere because it contains the language centers of the brain for most people. In the vast majority of people, a large left middle cerebral artery (MCA) territory ischemic stroke will cause dysfunction of one or both of the language centers. This will produce either a non-fluent aphasia (injury to Broca's area in the frontal lobe), fluent aphasia (injury to Wernicke's area in the posterosuperior temporal lobe), or global aphasia (injury to both). Additionally, though impairment varies with infarct size, large left MCA territory ischemic infarcts also present with right arm greater than leg weakness with sensory deficits, right homonymous hemianopia, and a left gaze deviation.

Though an in-depth description of the CT finding of large MCA territory infarcts was provided in a previous riddle, it should also be noted that brightness on non-contrasted CT often represents blood products, which in the case of a stroke, most often means either a hemorrhagic stroke or hemorrhagic conversion of an ischemic stroke. It should also be noted that on the National Institute of Health Stroke Scale (NIH-SS), the scoring is significantly skewed toward signs and symptoms of left MCA territory strokes as damage to the language centers will impair how the patient communicates and responds to commands provided during the exam.

As is true in clinical neurology, different types of pathologies affecting the same area can manifest with the same deficits, so it is critical to remember that a large primary intracerebral hemorrhage (ICH) affecting the left hemisphere can mimic a large MCA territory infarct. Usually, these patients report a severe headache at onset and are severely hypertensive. A quick non-contrast head CT can easily differentiate between the two.

Although a left hemispheric ICH will most likely present with a left gaze deviation, just like a left MCA infarction, it can on very rare occasions present with a right gaze deviation (wrong-way eyes).

35

• • • • •

Chronic axial rigid,
Autoimmune disease amid,
Diffuse spasm, look fluid in,
For anti-GAD, amphiphysin.

Hint #1

Name was changed in 1991 to a more gender-neutral name.

Hint #2

High co-occurrence with gluten sensitivity.

Stiff Person Syndrome

Stiff person syndrome (SPS) is a rare disease with an unclear pathogenesis, which presents with muscle stiffness and spasms. Symptoms are usually progressive and begin with gradual, intermittent, mildly painful muscle spasms that primarily affect the lower extremities and paraspinal muscles. These localized spasms later increase in frequency and intensity, occasionally becoming so severe that they produce painful abnormal postures, disability, and even fractured bones. Spasms can also be highly susceptible to multiple triggers such as touch, loud noise, and even emotion, and typically resolve with sleep.

Stiff person syndrome is currently divided into three subtypes – classic, partial, and paraneoplastic. The classic form primarily affects trunk muscles, and subsequently affecting balance and gait. The partial form usually affects one limb, typically a leg and affects gait. The paraneoplastic form is clinically similar to the other two forms but is paraneoplastic in origin and the GAD65 antibodies are usually negative.

The majority of patients with SPS have anti-GAD antibodies. Needle EMG demonstrates continuous motor-unit activity that can be abolished with benzodiazepines.

Progressive encephalomyelitis with rigidity and myoclonus (PERM) is a rare condition, which is considered to be on the same spectrum as SPS. It clinically mimics but presents with a rapidly progressive encephalitis with profound myoclonus and usually has a bad prognosis. Some of the patients with PERM also have anti-GAD antibodies.

Treatment options include benzodiazepines and baclofen for more severe cases. Immunotherapy with IVIG can also be used in patients who do not respond to benzodiazepines and baclofen.

36

• • • • •

Patient pacing round the room,
Repeat attacks quick to resume,
Miosis, tears, and headache ease,
With oxygen and CCBs.

Hint #1

Often describe a sharp/stabbing-type pain.

Hint #2

Pain attacks are grouped.

Cluster Headache

Well known for their excruciating pain, cluster headaches are a relatively rare and severe form of primary headache disorder, and more specifically, a type of trigeminal autonomic cephalgia. The pathogenesis of cluster headaches is thought to be different from that of migraine as PET scans have shown the activation of the posterior hypothalamus during cluster headache attacks, as opposed to the mesencephalic structures that become activated in migraine attacks. The involvement of the hypothalamus is thought to play a part in the circadian periodicity of the attacks experienced by individuals with cluster headaches.

Those with cluster headache often report headache attacks that develop over minutes, occur 1–8 times per day, typically "clustering" at certain times of day, and lasting 15 minutes to 3 hours. These attacks are often described as "sharp" and "stabbing," sometimes "boring" unilateral (usually affecting the same side each attack). During these attacks the patient will also experience rhinorrhea and lacrimation on the side of the headache. Cluster headaches often happen at night, waking patients from their sleep, with pain so severe that the patient is left sleeplessly pacing around the room, as opposed to the still and quiet sought by individuals with migraine.

Development and timing of cluster headaches are key differentiators of cluster headaches from migraine and other headache syndromes as, unlike migraine, cluster headaches tend to "cluster," with many severe headaches occurring at certain times of the day. Cluster headaches can also be differentiated from other forms of severe rapid headaches such as short-lasting unilateral neuralgiform attacks with conjunctival injection and tearing (SUNCT) syndrome and secondary causes of rapid headache like subarachnoid hemorrhage (SAH) and reversible cerebral vasoconstriction syndrome (RCVS) as peak headache intensity during cluster headaches is reached in minutes, not in seconds as in SUNCT, SAH, and RCVS.

The treatment of an acute attack requires administration of oxygen via a nonrebreather mask for ~15 minutes. If the attack resolves, preventive therapy can be initiated. If not, other treatment options include triptans and intranasal lidocaine. The preventive treatment of choice for patients with frequent attacks is verapamil with or without a short course of steroids. For infrequent attacks, only steroids can be used. Other options include lithium, galcanezumab, and topiramate.

37

• • • • •

Headache, drowsy, fever, seizure,
Normal glucose, high lymphocyte,
Polymerase inhibitor,
If mesotemporal is bright.

Hint #1

Often hemorrhagic.

Hint #2

Commonly treated clinically rather than based on lab results.

HSV-1 Encephalitis

Herpes simplex virus type 1 (HSV-1) is the most common cause of sporadic encephalitis in the United States, and carries with it a ~20% mortality in treated individuals, and ~70% in those untreated. Symptoms of HSV-1 encephalitis commonly include mental status changes, focal neurological deficits (hemiparesis, aphasia, and visual defects), headache, and seizures.

In the case of possible HSV-1 encephalitis, unless it is contraindicated, a lumbar puncture should be performed as CSF often shows a lymphocytic pleocytosis, elevated protein, with a high opening pressure, in the setting of normal to low CSF glucose. These values, however, can vary greatly in immunocompromised patients such as those with organ transplant or HIV/AIDS. CSF studies will often also show xanthochromia in correspondence with elevated RBCs. If encephalitis is suspected, HSV PCR, in addition to a complete CSF infectious workup should be performed, though it is often negative early in the course.

Neuroimaging for encephalitis typically begins with a non-contrasted CT of the head. In the case of HSV-1 encephalitis, which has a predilection for infecting and causing hemorrhage and edema in the medial temporal and orbitofrontal lobes, these areas may appear hyperdense (bright) on non-contrasted CT. If possible, follow-up neuroimaging with contrasted MRI is recommended, which usually shows a characteristic unilateral T2/FLAIR hyperintensity in the medial temporal, insular, and inferior frontal lobes, with or without hemorrhage on gradient echo series. On EEG, focal periodic lateralized epileptiform discharges (LPDs) are commonly seen.

Any patient who presents with encephalopathy and new onset focal seizures must be empirically treated with acyclovir, while waiting for a lumbar puncture. Delayed treatment can lead to poor prognosis. Symptomatic seizures are treated with anti-seizure medications. These patients often develop chronic epilepsy.

38

• • • • •

Psychiatric comorbid,
Two-third of fifth nerves of brain,
Sodium channel blockers,
For side-locked, shock-like, not tooth pain.

Hint #1

Pain is often described as sharp and shooting.

Hint #2

Not a movement disorder though used to be called "tic."

Trigeminal Neuralgia

Previously called tic douloureux, trigeminal neuralgia (TN) is the most common cause of neurogenic facial pain. Those with TN usually complain of sudden, superficial, sharp, stabbing, or burning unilateral facial pain over the V2 and/or V3 territories of the trigeminal nerve (maxilla and mandible). These attacks usually last seconds and can be triggered by touching or moving the affected area of the face. Unlike most other headache and facial pain syndromes, during TN attacks, the highest intensity of pain is experienced instantaneously at the onset of the attack, and resolves in seconds, with no symptoms between attacks, which are typically experienced daily for weeks to months prior to spontaneous remission for months to years.

Trigeminal neuralgia can be idiopathic, but it is imperative to look for secondary causes. In younger patients, especially women, multiple sclerosis is an important cause of TN. Hence, MRI of brain with and without contrast must be performed in these patients and history of other transient neurological symptoms must be elicited. Other secondary causes of TN include aberrant vascular loops, causing mechanical compression of the trigeminal nerve close to its entry into pons. If no clear demyelinating lesions are seen on MRI, then vascular imaging like magnetic resonance angiography (MRA) must be performed.

The first-line treatment options for TN include carbamazepine and oxcarbazepine. Other options include valproate, lamotrigine, phenytoin, and baclofen. For patients who are refractory to medical management and have an aberrant vascular loop causing TN, microvascular decompressive surgery is recommended. Gamma knife radiosurgery and rhizotomy are also available as surgical options.

39

• • • • •

Subclinically often present,
Due to protein so wrongly bent,
Black spots best seen on GRE,
With older age and APO-E.

Hint #1

Use caution with antiplatelet and anticoagulant medications.

Hint #2

Usually cortically predominant.

Cerebral Amyloid Angiopathy

Cerebral amyloid angiopathy (CAA) is a chronic microvasculopathy caused by the misfolding of amyloid beta-peptide in the brain and deposition of the misfolded amyloid in the walls of small and medium cerebral blood vessels. Though the exact pathogenesis of the CAA is unknown, and most cases are thought to be sporadic, hereditary CAA does exist and involves the possession of the β-amyloid precursor protein (β-APP) on chromosome 21, which is thought to be responsible for the misfolding of the protein. Additionally, those with APO-ϵ4 allele(s) have been found to have higher rates of CAA occurrence, and CAA is much more common in the elderly.

Due to the accumulation of misfolded structural proteins in the walls of cortical blood vessels with CAA, blood vessels become fragile and are much more prone to rupture, which subsequently leads to lobar hemorrhage. On neuroimaging, usually with non-contrasted CT and subsequent MRI, the lobar hemorrhages caused by CAA can often be seen in the parietal and occipital lobes, though they can be found anywhere cortically. Understandably, CAA and resulting lobar hemorrhage(s) can produce presenting symptoms of focal neurological deficit, altered mental status, headache, and seizure, depending on the size and location of the hemorrhage(s). Though large lobar hemorrhages can often be seen easily on CT, gradient-echo MRI series is preferred to delineate the severity and distribution of the characteristic diffuse cortically distributed microhemorrhages that accumulate over years and are often clinically silent. Additionally, given its association with cerebral amyloid deposition and APO-ϵ4, these individuals also commonly have symptoms of both vascular and nonvascular dementia.

40

. . . . .

Numbness, foot drop, hammer toe,
Pes cavus in families show,
Progress to hands in those who,
Duplicate PMP22.

Hint #1

Think "onion bulb."

Hint #2

Dx requires EMG.

Charcot–Marie Tooth

Charcot–Marie Tooth (CMT) is the most common type of hereditary peripheral neuropathy known as hereditary motor and sensory neuropathy (HMSN). These individuals typically experience a gradual distal lower extremity weakness and sensory loss over years, which results in symmetric distal lower extremity atrophy, foot drop, hammertoes, and pes cavus foot deformities. Distal upper extremity weakness and numbness will often occur as the lower extremity symptoms progress up the knees.

The most common subtype of CMT is CMT type 1 (HMSN 1) accounting for ~60% of all inherited peripheral neuropathies. It is caused by a mutation in the gene called peripheral myelin protein 22 (PMP22). The most common mutation is duplication. On the other hand, the deletion of PMP22 leads to a different phenotype known as hereditary neuropathy with pressure palsy. Another, clinically similar but often more severe and earlier onset subtype of CMT is CMT-1B, which is known for producing an "onion bulb" myelin appearance on nerve biopsy due to the repetitive demyelination and remyelination, and produces palpably enlarged peripheral nerves. Other subtypes of CMT are differentiated based on their inheritance pattern and/or the age of onset with CMT-X being passed via X-linked recessive inheritance; CMT-2 being inherited via autosomal dominant or recessive and often presenting in the patients' teens; CMT-3 (also called Dejerine-Sottas Disease) being inherited in the same way as CMT-2, but presents in infancy; and CMT-4 being passed by autosomal recessive inheritance and presents in childhood.

The diagnosis of CMT must be suspected in patients with very slowly progressive symptoms since childhood and the characteristic deformities of pes cavus and hammertoes.

The next step in the diagnostic process typically involves NCS/EMG. Typical NCS findings include prolonged conduction velocities and prolonged latencies. As opposed to cases of acquired demyelination (e.g., AIDP, CIDP), conduction blocks and temporal dispersion are not seen. Genetic testing with next-generation sequencing must be performed to identify the culprit gene. Current treatment options are only supportive.

41

• • • • •

Weakness fatigue, and numbness too,
Some vision loss, cannot pee on cue,
Some progress and some remit,
McDonald and Dawson know it.

Hint #1

The answer is separated by time and space.

Hint #2

Prevalence increase with latitude.

Multiple Sclerosis

Multiple sclerosis (MS) is an autoimmune, neuroinflammatory demyelinating disease, with a propensity for onset in middle-aged women, although it can occur in men and is rarely diagnosed in those above 65 years. Other risk modifiers include distance from the equator, as prevalence increases with greater latitudes. This is thought to be associated with low vitamin D, which also results in a predisposition to develop multiple sclerosis. Additionally twin studies show that there is some extent of a genetic component of MS as concordant rates of acquiring MS in monozygotic twins were 30% as opposed to 5% in dizygotic twins.

The pathogenesis remains poorly understood, though the histology of MS is relatively well known. Patients with MS develop episodic and progressive inflammatory plaques primarily in the periventricular white matter, optic nerves, spinal cord, and corpus callosum. Histologically, these plaques are composed of focal inflammatory cell infiltration (lymphocytes and macrophages), and myelin and oligodendrocyte loss, with preservation of axons.

The onset of MS symptoms is often acute though can be insidious and vary greatly in severity. Most commonly these patients first experience one or more of some sort of sensory disturbance, motor weakness, vision loss or diplopia, or ataxia. Not uncommonly, patients also report preceding symptoms of fatigue or headache. Sensory disturbances experienced can be hypoesthesias, paresthesias, or dysesthesias, as well as a squeezing sensation around their truck or limb. Motor deficits can often develop over a course of days or only apparent after strenuous exercise, though may be acute onset. The acute vision loss, optic neuritis, which is often experienced as the first symptom, can present as slowly progressive (over days) partial or full vision loss, usually unilateral. This can present as an isolated event or concomitant with other signs and symptoms and is caused by focal inflammation of the optic nerve. Diplopia in MS is often caused by demyelinating plaque formation in the medial longitudinal fasciculus producing a condition called internuclear ophthalmoplegia (INO) resulting in impaired adduction of the ipsilateral eye as well as compensatory nystagmus of the abducting eye on attempted contralateral horizontal gaze.

The diagnosis of MS is made using the 2017 McDonald criteria. The two critical principles in the diagnostic process are "dissemination in space" and "dissemination in time." Dissemination in space (DIS) is defined by identification of clinical attacks affecting different CNS sites or by evidence of MRI lesions affecting at least two typical MS sites. Dissemination in time (DIT) is defined by different clinical attacks separated by time or by the presence of contrast enhancing and nonenhancing lesions on MRI. Criteria for both DIS and DIT must be met for the diagnosis. The presence of CSF oligoclonal bands can be used as a supportive criterion.

Typical MRI findings include T2/FLAIR hyperintensities in the periventricular white matter (Dawson's fingers), juxtacortical, and/ or subcortical white matter. Spinal cord hyperintensities can also be seen with these modalities indicating the involvement of the spinal cord in MS. Over time, progressive plaque formation usually results in significant cerebral and spinal cord atrophy.

The most common phenotype of MS is relapsing–remitting, which is characterized by clearly defined attacks, interrupted by periods of remission.

The differential diagnoses include NMOSD (neuromyelitis optica spectrum disorder), ADEM (acute demyelinating encephalomyelitis), and MOGAD (myelin oligodendrocyte glycoprotein antibody-associated disease).

Acute clinical attacks are treated with high dose steroids and plasma exchange. Long-term treatment consists of disease-modifying agents such as dimethyl fumarate, fingolimod, siponimod, teriflunomide, natalizumab, ocrelizumab, rituximab, or ofatumumab.

42

• • • • •

Dysfunction in the short term made,
Memories anterograde,
Focal defic-its or seizures nay,
Memory comes back less than one day.

Hint #1

Believed by some to involve cortical spreading depression.

Hint #2

Confusion and disorientation are the main symptoms.

Transient Global Amnesia

In individuals with transient global amnesia (TGA), acute inability to create new memories (anterograde amnesia) and disorientation are the primary symptoms; however, some often have a degree of retrograde amnesia as well. In ~50% of those with TGA, the onset of symptoms is often during times of emotional or physical stress. During an episode of TGA, there is no change in alertness or loss of consciousness, or changes in any other cognitive or neurological domains, and episodes usually last from 4-24 hours.

The exact cause and pathogenesis of TGA is unknown; however, some studies implicate the CA1 region of the hippocampus and some theorize that the effects of TGA may be due to the "spreading depression" phenomena, which is also thought to be the cause of migraine auras. There appears to be a higher prevalence in those who also experience migraines. Transient global amnesia is much more common in those greater than 50 years of age. Usually, given the patients' profound anxiety and anterograde amnesia, the diagnosis of TGA requires the help of a witness to confirm that there was no head trauma or seizure-like activity at or near symptom onset. In addition to acute transient anterograde amnesia, these patients may have trouble remembering other social and historical information such as where they work, who their family members are, or where they live, though they retain the ability to follow complex commands and complete all activities of daily living. During TGA the patient has full awareness of their identity.

After the TGA episode has passed, the patient often remains amnestic to events that occurred during and shortly before the episode. There is no definitive diagnostic tool available for TGA; however, neuroimaging, urine toxicology, and the event description by a witness can help to rule out other causes such as stroke or seizure. Some studies have shown that MRI may show a DWI signal in the medial temporal lobes during an episode. The recurrence of TGA is ~5-10%.

The major differential characteristics for TGA include migrainous aura, epileptic seizures, and stroke. These can be relatively easily differentiated by taking a detailed history. There is no specific treatment, just reassurance, for TGA. If the episodes recur in a stereotypical fashion, the diagnosis of epilepsy must be considered.

43

• • • • •

Older woman, painful jaw,
Granulomas, vessel flaw,
If disc swells, things hard to see,
Then steroids quick, and biopsy.

Hint #1

Do not chew on this question too long. It might start to hurt.

Hint #2

Associated with polymyalgia rheumatic.

Temporal Arteritis

Also called *giant cell arteritis* (GCA), temporal arteritis is the most common systemic vasculitis in those greater than 50. It mainly affects large- and medium-sized arteries. Specifically, Caucasian women of northern European descent are the most commonly affected. The histopathology demonstrates granulomatous organization of CD4 cells and macrophages with the formation of giant cells. The carotid arteries are very commonly affected. Patients with GCA also often experience symptoms of headache and jaw claudication. Diplopia can also occur with GCA due to ischemia of the extraocular muscles. But the most significant symptom is transient visual loss, which is caused by the vasculopathy extending into the arteries supplying the retina and the optic nerve. The typical presentation is an acute complete or partial monocular painless visual loss. Although the visual symptoms can be transient, this should prompt an urgent investigation and treatment because of the significant risk of permanent visual loss. Though less common, ischemic strokes can also occur with GCA due to the involvement of the internal carotid arteries and rarely vertebral arteries.

On exam, in addition to the signs listed above, patients often also experience tenderness to palpation over the temporal arteries, which may feel thickened to the examiner. Fundoscopy demonstrates optic disc edema with early onset pallor (pallid edema), contrasted to the hyperemic disc edema of non-arteritic ischemic optic neuropathy. This finding of pallid disc edema (chalky-white appearance) in a patient above 50 years of age is almost exclusively seen in temporal arteritis. Bloodwork will show elevated inflammatory markers with erythrocyte sedimentation rate (ESR) >50 mm/h in most patients, or an elevated C-reactive protein in the setting of a normal ESR. Careful ophthalmological evaluation for optic disc edema is required in these patients. Though vessel imaging can be helpful, the gold standard for diagnosis is a temporal artery biopsy.

If GCA is suspected, empiric treatment with high-dose steroids should be started immediately, regardless of the timing of the temporal artery biopsy. After initial treatment with high dose IV steroids, maintenance therapy with high dose oral prednisone 60 mg daily must be continued for one week, following which it is tapered very slowly over 52 weeks. In some patients, steroid sparing agents like tocilizumab can also be used.

44

• • • • •

Seizures and altered mentation,
Noninfectious constellation CSF,
With high white cell,
In fluid antibodies dwell.

Hint #1

Consider treating with plasma exchange or IVIG.

Hint #2

Lymphocytic pleocytosis.

Autoimmune Encephalitis

Autoimmune encephalitis (AI) is a relatively newly defined group of noninfectious, immune-mediated inflammatory conditions of the brain parenchyma. First described in the 1960s, AI was originally found to be a paraneoplastic limbic encephalitis due to small cell lung cancer. A decade later research proved that this condition is caused by antibodies directed against either intracellular onconeuronal antigens, for example, anti-Hu or against the neuronal surface antigens, for example, anti-N-methyl-D-aspartate receptor (NMDAR). Most of the classic paraneoplastic autoimmune encephalitides belong to the former category.

Understandably, symptomology of autoimmune encephalitides varies widely; however, for most cases, patients present with days to weeks of progressive lethargy, confusion, personality change, and seizures with or without the involvement of the cranial nerves or spinal cord. Changes in personality and cognition will be much more prominent in patients with autoimmune limbic encephalitis. In cases of paraneoplastic AI, the symptoms of AI often precede the discovery of cancer, with ~50% of paraneoplastic autoimmune encephalitides occurring in the setting of lung cancer, ~20% occurring with testicular cancer, and 8% occurring with breast cancer.

Though MRI usually shows limbic encephalitis as a unilateral or bilateral T2/FLAIR hyperintensity in the mesial temporal lobes, broadly, AI as a larger group of diseases can be seen as hyperintensities anywhere in the brain. If AI is suspected, additional imaging should be pursued in the attempt to find a neoplastic cause as well as a lumbar puncture to both rule out other forms of encephalitis and look for causal antibodies. Many serum and CSF antibody tests are now available for the investigation of AI antibodies.

Specific antibody testing must only be performed if and when the clinical suspicion is high. Both serum and CFS samples must be sent at the same time. The treatment must be aggressive and options include steroids, IVIG, rituximab, and cyclophosphamide. Paraneoplastic AI cases often do not respond very well to immuno-therapy, especially those associated with onconeural antibodies. The best way to treat such cases is to find the cancer and treat it. For non-paraneoplastic AI, especially those with surface anti-bodies, immunotherapy works well.

45

● ● ● ● ●

Proximal and distal weak,
Rimmed vacuolated fibers seek,
Plus eosinophils display,
With positive CN1A.

Hint #1

Commonly present with grip weakness.

Hint #2

Painless weakness and wasting.

Inclusion Body Myositis

Though inclusion body myositis (IBM) shares many of the same qualities and characteristics of other types of inflammatory myopathies, its onset is usually later in life (>50 years) and more often presents unilaterally than polymyositis (PM) and dermatomyositis (DM). Inclusion body myositis is the most common inflammatory myopathy in patients above 50 years of age.

The pattern of signs and symptoms of IBM helps distinguish it from PM as IBM progresses much more slowly (months to years) and, unlike PM and DM, which present primarily with symmetrical proximal muscle weakness, IBM presents with asymmetric, distal, painless muscle weakness in the wrist, fingers, and feet, in addition to proximal limb weakness. The most characteristic examination findings are weakness and atrophy of quadriceps and forearm flexor muscles. Coexisting autoimmune diseases are also seen in ~15% of those with IBM.

Creatinine kinase has low diagnostic quality for IBM as CK can range from normal to 10 times the upper limit of normal. Similarly, myositis-specific antibodies are rarely present in the absence of co-occurring autoimmune disease. Anti-cytosolic 5′-nucleotidase 1A (cN1A) can be found in one third to two thirds of patients with IBM, though this is not specific to IBM nor to acute disease. Investigation with EMG and NCS usually shows spontaneous activity, and other typical myopathic characteristics and muscle biopsy can show a variety of atrophy, necrosis, endomysial inflammation, rimmed vacuoles, and β-amyloid-containing eosinophilic inclusion bodies. The β-amyloid deposition has led to recent questioning of IBM being more of a myodegenerative process rather than an autoimmune pathology.

Treatment is mainly supportive. Glucocorticoids and other immunosuppressive medications do not have any clear benefit; hence, most experts do not recommend using them.

46

• • • • •

Second most common found in kid,
Mostly cerebellar mid,
Nausea, vomit, head is aching,
Obstructed flow dilation making.

Hint #1

The answer can often be found sagitally.

Hint #2

Arises from primitive neuroectoderm.

Medulloblastoma

Prior to the reclassification of tumors by molecular parameters in 2016, medulloblastomas were called "primitive neuroectodermal tumors." Medulloblastomas are the most common embryonic tumor, and after astrocytoma, they are the second most common type of pediatric brain tumor (most common malignant pediatric brain tumor). Though medulloblastoma is more commonly found in adolescent boys than girls, it can also be found in young and middle-aged adults.

Signs and symptoms of medulloblastomas slightly differ from many other tumor types as it is not often associated with focal weakness or seizure, but rather with those of obstructive hydrocephalus such as nausea, vomiting, and headache. Given its predilection for the posterior fossa and parenchymal damage to the cerebellum, ataxia is also commonly seen.

On neuroimaging, medulloblastomas are usually seen as a well-defined cerebellar hyperdense mass on CT, which is hyperintense on T2/FLAIR MRI with heterogenous contrast enhancement on T1 Gad sequence. It is often located close to the midline in the roof of the fourth ventricle. Medulloblastomas are well documented to disseminate via CSF if found, and further imaging of the entire neuroaxis should be completed.

Based on the underlying molecular genetics, medulloblastomas are classified into four groups – SHH (sonic hedgehog) pathway, WNT (wingless-related integration site) pathway, group 3, and group 4. These groups have different genetics, different histological features, and different prognoses.

Treatment is aimed at first reducing the intracranial pressure and relieving the hydrocephalus, if present. This usually involves a shunt placement. Maximal surgical resection of the tumor is very important. After surgery, radiation therapy is provided to the entire neuroaxis and especially to the primary tumor site. Chemotherapy is also used in high-risk cases. The prognosis varies depending upon the molecular group. The highest five-year survival is seen in the WNT group and the lowest survival is in group 3.

47

• • • • •

Droopy eyelid, trouble sweating,
And Slurr'ed speech, vertigo getting,
Numbness on same side of face,
Opposite body numb displays.

Hint #1

Think brainstem.

Hint #2

Still stumped? Ask Dr. Horner.

Lateral Medullary Syndrome

Also known as "Wallenberg syndrome," lateral medullary syndrome is a common brainstem stroke syndrome and is caused by ischemia of the dorsolateral medulla, which is nourished by the posterior inferior cerebellar artery (PICA), which comes off the vertebral artery. In the majority of cases, the culprit vessel is the vertebral artery itself causing artery-to-artery embolism. This vascular occlusion produces a wedge-shaped infarct in the dorsolateral medulla, posterior to the inferior olivary nucleus. Though it was first described by Swiss physician Gaspard Vieusseux in 1808, it was later explained in more detail by German neurologist Adolf Wallenberg in 1895, whose name this syndrome still carries.

The typical signs and symptoms include imbalance, vertigo, nystagmus hoarseness, and dysphagia. However, the complete list of signs, symptoms, and relevant clinical anatomy is given below, as outlined by Canadian neurologist Dr. Charles Miller Fisher in 1961:

1. Vestibular nuclei: vertigo, nystagmus, oscillopsia
2. Spinothalamic tract: impaired perception of contralateral pain and temperature.
3. Descending sympathetic tract: ipsilateral ptosis, miosis, and anhidrosis (Horner syndrome).
4. CNs 9 and 10: hoarse voice, dysphagia, ipsilateral vocal cord and palatal paralysis, hiccups, and reduced gag reflex.
5. Utricular pathway: ocular tilt reaction with skew deviation. The eye ipsilateral to the lesion is hypotropic and the contralateral eye is hypertropic. This is associated with contralesional torsional nystagmus.
6. Inferior cerebellar peduncle, olivocerebellar and spinocerebellar fibers, and restiform body: ipsilateral ataxia and lateropulsive sensation. This is also associated with saccadic ipsipulsion.

7. CN 5 nucleus and descending tract: ipsilateral facial numbness or pain (burning).
8. Nucleus solitarius: loss of taste.
9. Nucleus gracilis and nucleus cuneatus (rare): ipsilateral sensory defect.

There is typically no weakness associated with this syndrome because of relative sparing of the more ventral and medial corticospinal tract. If the lesion extends into the corticospinal tract prior to decussation, it will be associated with contralateral weakness. This variant of Wallenberg syndrome is called Babinski–Nageotte syndrome. Rarely, the Wallenberg syndrome is associated with ipsilateral weakness because of extension of the lesion into corticospinal tract after decussation. This variant is called Opalski syndrome.

48

• • • • •

Abnormal vessels, CNS,
Notably capillary-less,
Tangles of high and low pressure,
Embolize/remove to cure.

Hint #1

Does the term "nidus" help?

Hint #2

Commonly present with cerebral hemorrhage.

Arteriovenous Malformation

An arteriovenous malformation (AVM) is a focal area of abnormally tangled arteries and veins within and around the brain or spinal cord. The arterial and venous vessels of the AVM connect with one another, with continuous flow, and are void of an intermediary capillary bed, producing direct arteriovenous shunting at the center of the AVM called the nidus.

Because of the abnormal hemodynamics in the AVM, hemorrhage is common with ~50% of patients presenting with intraparenchymal, subarachnoid, or intraventricular hemorrhage. Signs and symptoms of AVMs often include seizures, headaches, and focal neurological deficits; however, they are often asymptomatic and found on neuroimaging incidentally. The yearly risk of an initial first hemorrhage for someone with an AVM is 1–4%, and after an initial hemorrhage, the yearly risk of rehemorrhaging increases significantly to 1–18% depending on many factors including the size of the nidus and the location of the AVM, as well as modifiable risk factors such as tobacco use, illicit drug use, and hypertension.

Whether a patient requires surgical intervention or not is determined by multiple factors in addition to the prior history of bleeding. The Spetzler–Martin grading scale incorporates the size of the AVM, location (eloquent vs. non-eloquent area), and deep venous drainage.

Surgical treatment options include microsurgical excision for grade 1 or 2 lesions. Stereotactic radiosurgery can also be used.

49

• • • • •

Confused and feet are stuck to floor,
And widely space, continence poor,
No obstruction, and normal flow,
Remove some fluid, watch him go.

Hint #1

Looking for high pressure? Won't find it here.

Hint #2

Stick to the clues like a magnet.

Normal Pressure Hydrocephalus

The pathogenesis of idiopathic normal pressure hydrocephalus (NPH) is poorly understood and even its existence has been contested. Normal pressure hydrocephalus is a chronic form of hydrocephalus (excessive fluid accumulation in the brain), which unlike acute hydrocephalus has a normal intracranial fluid pressure. Also, unlike acute hydrocephalus, in NPH there is no obstruction in the CSF flow pathway, earning NPH its other name, communicating hydrocephalus. Understanding the exact mechanism of NPH has been difficult given often co-occurring neurodegenerative diseases, particularly dementias.

Most commonly, those with NPH exhibit a chronic progressive "magnetic" and apraxic-type gait disturbance characterized by difficulty lifting their feet off the ground as well as a "freezing" phenomenon similar to that found in Parkinson disease. However, unlike Parkinsonian gait, those with NPH usually have wide-based gait and externally rotated feet. Those with NPH commonly also have symptoms of incontinence though may only have urinary urgency and frequency. Lastly, the often-cited triad of signs of NPH are (1) gait disturbance; (2) urinary incontinence; and (3) cognitive impairment. A subcortical type of progressive dementia is often seen as the last of the three symptoms to develop, in which bradyphrenia, forgetfulness, and apathy are most prominent.

Other than helping to exclude other causes, bloodwork is often unhelpful in the diagnosis of NPH. Neuroimaging with CT or MRI showing central ventricular enlargement that is out of proportion to the surrounding cerebral atrophy is required for diagnosis. Also helpful in diagnosis is the lumbar puncture, which in the case of NPH will show normal CSF pressure and often improvement in gait speed after large volume (35–50 mL) CSF removal using a recorded 8–10 meter walk test. The effects of CSF removal on gait speed usually last for just hours. Similarly, given the chronic nature of the hydrocephalus, some clinicians choose to remove more CSF over a longer period of time (~10 mL/hr over 3–5 days) using more invasive techniques involving lumbar drains and catheters, though these modalities carry with them higher complication risks.

The existence of NPH as a distinct clinical entity has been debated. A review of multiple NPH studies evaluating the efficacy of shunting has clearly demonstrated that the "benefits" of CSF shunting are short-lasting. A study also demonstrated that a significant proportion of patients diagnosed with NPH have pathological evidence of Alzheimer disease at the time of shunting. It has been postulated that instead of idiopathic NPH, this condition must be referred to as neurodegenerative NPH, and that this communicating form of hydrocephalus earlier in the disease course is simply a manifestation of neurodegeneration. There is also no evidence to suggest that the point at which CSF shunting is performed prevents the "progression" of the disease. Experts recommend that it is high time to conduct a randomized clinical trial with longer follow-up to truly evaluate if CSF shunting helps such patients.

50

· · · · ·

Slower onset, less severe,
Compromised patients know and fear,
Low glucose, high lymphocyte,
Headache, stiff neck, and dura bright.

Fungal Meningitis

Fungal meningitis is far rarer than viral and bacterial meningitis and is more commonly seen in immunocompromised patients. The most common fungal pathogen is *Cryptococcus neoformans*, followed by *Candida* species, then *Coccidioides*, and then *Histoplasma*. In immunosuppressed patients, particularly those with AIDS and a CD4 count <200, cryptococcal meningitis infections represent a reemergence of an existing infection, and are a large contributor to HIV-related death. In addition to those with AIDS, those who have undergone an organ transplant, or with malignancy, or with uncontrolled diabetes mellitus, or on chemotherapeutics are also at a higher risk of CNS fungal infections.

The risk of acquiring specific species of fungal meningitis can change based on environmental exposure and other pre-existing medical conditions, such as spores in dirt (*Coccidioides* in southwest USA and Mexico; *Aspergillius* and *Histoplasma* in the Ohio and Mississippi river valley, USA), bird or bat feces (*Cryptococcus*), IV-drug use or poorly controlled blood sugar (*Mucor*), and chronic antibiotic use (*Candida*).

Patients with fungal meningitis most often first experience a chronic headache that progressively worsens over weeks to months, which is often accompanied by a progressive encephalopathy in ~50% of these patients. The typical meningeal signs of nuchal rigidity and fever are often less predominant in fungal meningitis.

Cerebrospinal fluid analysis is required to establish a diagnosis and will typically show a characteristic lymphocyte predominant pleocytosis with low glucose and high protein. There is, however, variability in these CSF values as in the cases of *Candida*, *Histoplasma*, *Aspergilus*, and *Blastomycosis*, and a neutrophilic predominance can be seen. In addition to CSF analysis with fungal assays and culture, if fungal meningitis is suspected, India ink staining will show characteristic round, budding, encapsulated cells. In cases where fungal meningitis is found, patients should be further investigated for malignancy or an underlying immunocompromising state.

Neuroimaging with contrasted MRI will almost always show meningeal enhancement, with predilection for the basilar meninges. It can also show obstructive hydrocephalus due to direct fugal blockage or ependymitis. In the case of candidal meningitis, co-occurrence of multiple, diffuse, hemorrhagic, ring-shaped micro-abscesses can be seen.

The treatment of fungal meningitis mainly involves liposomal amphotericin in combination with flucytosine. After several weeks of amphotericin therapy, oral fluconazole can be used. Other agents that can be used include voriconazole, posaconazole, and caspofungin.

51

• • • • •

Spores in soil, come within,
Tissue necrosis, spasmed grin,
If progress will backward bend,
Debridement and toxoid will end.

Hint #1

Maybe try the spatula test.

Hint #2

Remember to periodically renew your immunization.

Tetanus

Tetanus is caused by the neurotoxin *tetanospasmin*, which is produced by the Gram-positive, anaerobic bacillus *Clostridium tetani*. The spores from *C. tetani* are ubiquitous in soil worldwide and most often enter through wound tissue, either traumatically or by inoculation of a pre-existing wound. In countries with poor access to vaccination and sterile medical care, it is a known complication of birthing. After wound tissue necrosis begins, giving the bacteria an environment to germinate and produce tetanospasmin, the neurotoxin then enters peripheral nerves, moving proximally to the spinal cord and brainstem. Ultimately, tetanospasmin creates excessive motor neuron discharges by blocking inhibitory interneurons.

Symptoms of tetanus are often delayed as there is typically a 1–3-week incubation period between inoculation and symptoms. The earliest signs of tetanus are usually trismus (lockjaw) as well as paraspinal and neck stiffness with a characteristic back-extended posture called *opisthotonos* and facial muscle stiffness giving the patient an eerie grin called *risus sardonicus*. Patients with tetanus also experience "tetanospasms," which are painful tonic spasms that can be triggered by light touch and occur spontaneously. Patients also often experience asphyxia and dysphagia due to laryngeal, diaphragm, and pharyngeal muscle spasms. Tetanospasmin can also produce dysfunction of the autonomic nervous system, resulting in diaphoresis, fever, cardiac dysrhythmias, and large blood pressure variation. Tetanospasmin has no direct effects on mentation.

Neuroimaging, bloodwork, and CSF analysis are only helpful in ruling out other causes, and unfortunately, *C. tetani* cannot be cultured from a wound. Though many of the signs of tetanus are easily observable, the signs of trismus can be elicited by the spatula test, which is positive when masseter spasm is elicited upon touching the oropharynx with a tongue blade or "spatula."

Treatment is mainly supportive and requires intensive care in a hospital. Wound debridement is important. Antibiotics like metronidazole and penicillin G are also used. The bound toxin cannot be neutralized but removing unbound toxin is known to improve the outcome. The agent of choice is human tetanus immune globulin.

52

• • • • •

Increased pressure, clot within,
Dull headache first to begin,
Focal signs may later be,
Imperfect flow on MRV.

Hint #1

More common in pregnancy and other hypercoagulable states.

Hint #2

Look out for elevated ICP.

Cerebral Venous Sinus Thrombosis

Cerebral venous sinus thrombosis (CVST) is characterized by a thrombus that forms in the cerebral venous sinuses and is most often spoken about in terms of the progressive, dull, pressure-type holocephalic headache it produces. Though women immediately postpartum are at the highest risk of developing CVST, young women who smoke in addition to taking oral contraception medications are at particularly high risk compared to the average population. The most common venous sinus involved in CVST is the superior sagittal sinus. Complications of CVST extend far beyond headache as increased intracranial pressure, cerebral edema, subarachnoid hemorrhage, alterations in consciousness, and papilledema commonly occur depending on severity and location.

The imaging modality of choice is MR venography using gadolinium. In patients where MR imaging is contraindicated, CT venography can be used as well. Treatment requires anticoagulation. Even if there is hemorrhage associated with the venous thrombosis, anticoagulation must be continued.

53

• • • • •

If pressure pain that's worse with lying,
And modified Dandy complying,
In overweight females exhibit,
Carbonic anhydrase inhibit.

Hint #1

Can result in optic disc edema.

Hint #2

Position-dependent headache.

Idiopathic Intracranial Hypertension

Idiopathic intracranial hypertension (IIH) is a syndrome caused by increased intracranial pressure without a mass lesion. In the past, IIH has been known by many names since being first discovered by German internist and surgeon Heinrich Quincke in 1897, shortly after developing the lumbar puncture. Dr. Quincke first named IIH "meningitis serosa." Just a few years later in 1904, German neurologist Max Nonne first published the term *pseudo-tumor cerebri* after noticing that the symptoms of IIH were similar to those found in patients with intracranial masses. This was later termed *benign intracranial hypertension* by J. Foley in 1955 to avoid the connotation of malignancy to the general public; however, given the possibility of permanent vision loss in untreated cases, and thus not "benign," this name has fallen out of favor.

Though the exact pathophysiology of IIH is unknown, many propose that the increased intracranial pressure (ICP) in these cases is due to impairment in the resorption of CSF into the venous sinuses by arachnoid villi. Women are nine times more commonly effected by IIH than men, and it is much more commonly seen in overweight women who are from 20–44 years of age.

The most commonly reported symptom of IIH is headache. The headache in IIH is often described as a daily holocephalic, throbbing-type headache that is worse when lying down (better with standing), and often associated with nausea, vomiting, and most concerningly, visual disturbance. Of the visual disturbance symptoms, the earliest to develop is often the constriction of the visual fields. Also commonly reported in patients with IIH are horizontal diplopia and pulsatile tinnitus. Patients with known or suspected IIH should receive an advanced ophthalmological evaluation to look for optic disk edema, peripheral visual field constriction, and enlargement of the physiological blind spot.

The diagnostic criteria of IIH were first proposed by Walter Dandy in 1937, and later modified by J. Lawton Smith in 1985, and the new criteria were named the "modified-Dandy" criteria. This has been again modified a few times to our current accepted diagnostic criteria for IIH. In general, these patients will have an elevated ICP $\geq$ 25 cm H_2O with normal CSF composition, many of the symptoms listed above, and neuroimaging showing no structural lesion to explain an increased ICP or symptoms. A brain MRI will also show normal to small ventricle size and many patients with IIH have an empty sella. Interestingly, there is a high co-occurrence of transverse sinus stenosis in IIH compared to the general population.

Management options include low sodium diet with weight loss. For patients with or without vision loss, treatment with acetazolamide is recommended. For patients with severe vision loss, acetazolamide must be rapidly uptitrated while consulting for surgical options like CSF shunting or optic nerve sheath fenestration.

54

• • • • •

More in women with greater than three,
Cord segments affected and she,
Will have cells in her fluid galore,
Optic neuritis and AQP4.

Hint #1

Increased reflexes.

Hint #2

Think weakness and bowel/bladder issues.

Neuromyelitis Optica Spectrum Disorder

Also called Devic's disease, after French neurologist Eugene Devic who first discovered and described the disease in 1894, neuromyelitis optica (NMO) is a highly aggressive spectrum of neuroinflammatory disease characterized by recurrent attacks of myelitis and optic neuritis. Occurring more frequently in women than in men (3:1) and usually in adulthood, the optic neuritis of NMO can be bilateral or unilateral, and the myelitis associated with NMO is typically longitudinally extensive, stretching to at least three vertebral segments of the spinal cord continuously. Though the majority of neural injury of NMO is associated with the inflammation of the spinal cord and optic nerves, recent studies have shown that patients with NMO also often have involvement of the brain including the area postrema, which causes intractable nausea and vomiting, and the hypothalamus, which causes endocrinopathies. Also, lesions of the cerebral hemispheres can be seen, producing a host of possible symptoms from focal neurological deficits to seizures, though they can also be asymptomatic.

In addition to focal enhancement and swelling of the optic nerves and spinal cord seen on MRI, CSF analysis is also helpful in making the diagnosis. In cases of NMO, CSF will usually show a pleocytosis of >50 cells with a common neutrophil predominance and eosinophils present. Oligoclonal bands can be present but not in the majority of cases. Like many other neuroinflammatory diseases, NMO is highly associated with autoimmune diseases such as systemic lupus, Sjogren syndrome, and PANCA-associated vasculitides. Autoantibody against the water channel protein aquaporin-4 (AQP4) has been found to be present in ~70% of those with NMO, and the detection of AQP4 in serum is both highly specific for NMO cases and predicts a >50% risk relapse in one year if untreated. In seronegative cases of NMO, approximately 40% will be positive for anti-MOG antibodies, and the patients often experience a more severe and rapidly sequential course than experienced by those with only AQP4 positivity.

As opposed to multiple sclerosis, the pathophysiology of NMO is well understood and it has a clear biomarker. NMO is a type of astrocytopathy as these AQP4 channels are mainly present on astrocytes. Both MS and NMO can cause optic neuritis, but bilateral optic neuritis should raise suspicion for NMO. Similarly, both MS and NMO can cause myelitis but longitudinally extensive myelitis (LETM) is much more commonly seen in NMO. Any patient with suspected MS must be checked for AQP4 antibodies because the treatment of MS and NMO is different. The current US FDA-approved medications for NMO include eculizumab, inebilizumab, and satralizumab. Because these drugs are still very expensive, many physicians still prefer using rituximab.

55

• • • • •

Most common parasite in brain,
From Latin "seat," of swine domain,
Seizures come and cysts you'll see,
With travel, a scolex will be.

Neurocysticercosis

Neurocysticercosis (NNC) is caused by the larval form of the pork tapeworm *Taenia solium* and is the most common parasitic infection of the CNS worldwide. *Taenia* in particular is commonly endemic to Central and South America, India, Sub-Saharan Africa, and East Asia, and infections have become more common with the expansion of travel and immigration.

In short, humans become infected with the eggs of *T. solium* by ingesting raw or undercooked pork. After ingestion, the eggs hatch in the small intestine, producing oncospheres that pierce through the wall of the small intestine, move into the bloodstream, ending up settling in brain and eye tissue, as well as muscle and other organs. These oncospheres develop into cysts at their end destination tissue until, after several months, they begin to degenerate or are killed by local host inflammation, which ultimately produces a calcified granuloma. Though ~60% of those with NCC have parenchymal cysts, there exists an alternative extraparechymal variant of NCC called racemose NCC that produces multiple confluent cysts in the subarachnoid and ventricular spaces, causing CSF obstruction and having a "cluster-of-grapes" appearance on the MRI.

The primary symptoms of NCC are seizures, headache, and meningeal signs, though some cases remain asymptomatic and are discovered incidentally. Hydrocephalus can be severe and produce changes in consciousness, and retinal involvement can produce visual scotomas. Calcified and uncalcified cysts as well as a scolex (the hooked mouth-like end of the mature *T. solium*) can be seen on both CT and MRI.

Diagnosis does not require ELISA serology, though it is available. Analysis of CSF will often show a relative eosinophilia (>10% of WBC) with normal CSF protein and glucose. The diagnosis can be made by finding this histopathological evidence, finding subretinal cysts, or identifying a scolex on neuroimaging, along with travel to or ingestion of food from endemic areas.

Neurocysticercosis is the most common cause of focal epilepsy in the world. Treatment requires anti-seizure medications. For patients with viable and/or degenerating cysts seen on neuroimaging, treatment is with either albendazole or a combination of albendazole and praziquantel.

56

• • • • •

Seen in kids from birth to three,
Some can walk, some born floppy,
Weakness, wasting, some reflex none,
Mutation in SMN1.

Hint #1

Unsure, ask Werdnig or Hoffman.

Hint #2

Look no further than chromosome 5q11.

Spinal Muscular Atrophy

Spinal muscular atrophy (SMA) is a type of motor neuron disease that is autosomal recessive and is passed by mutation of the SMN1 (survival motor neuron 1) gene located at chromosome 5q11. Though SMA is divided into four subtypes (SMA 1-4) based on the severity and age of onset of symptoms, symptoms generally consist of subacute weakness and lower motor neuron signs in the absence of sensory or cognitive impairment. Postural tremor is very common, and the vast majority of these individuals have tongue fasciculations.

With symptom onset beginning at <6 months of age, and at times found at birth, SMA 1, also historically called Werdnig-Hoffman disease after they first described the disease in the 1890s, is the second leading cause of death from a recessively inherited disease, after cystic fibrosis. These babies are typically noted to be weak or "floppy" from birth. Hypotonia, muscle wasting, and respiratory muscle weakness are significant, and these infants typically die before the age of two due to respiratory failure or infection, and they never gain the ability to sit upright.

Symptom onset for SMA 2, also called chronic infantile SMA, is usually between 6 and 18 months. These children develop the ability to sit upright unsupported and often live into their twenties and thirties. In SMA 3, also called chronic juvenile SMA or Kugelberg-Welander disease, affected individuals develop much milder symptoms such as difficulty walking up stairs or other gait abnormalities, though they have normal life expectancies. SMA 4 is the adult-onset subtype of SMA in which symptom of difficulty walking and proximal limb weakness often begin in early adulthood.

Bloodwork will often show a very mildly elevated CK level, though usually <3 times the upper level of normal. Spontaneous activity as evidenced by fibrillations and positive sharp waves as well as motor unit action potentials with long duration, high amplitude, and reduced recruitment are seen on EMG. Definitive diagnosis is made by genetic testing showing SMN1 gene mutation. The variability in the clinical severity of different subgroups of SMA is determined by another gene called SMN2. With SMN1 gene mutation and loss of SMN protein synthesis, there is partial compensation provided by the SMN2 gene. The less the number of SMN2 copies available, the more severe the disease phenotype.

Other than supportive management, treatment options include antisense oligonucleotide (ASO) therapy such as nusinersen. These modify the splicing of the SMN2 gene to increase the production of SMN protein. Another treatment option is gene therapy administered via recombinant adeno-associated viral vector. This vector contains DNA coding for SMN protein. This drug is called onasemnogene abeparvovec.

57

• • • • •

Symmetric arms and shoulder jerks,
In teens when they see fireworks,
Morning clumsiness you'll see,
And often runs in family.

Hint #1

Keep these patients away from strobe lights.

Hint #2

Has however been reported from ages 8–26 years old.

183

Juvenile Myoclonic Epilepsy

A common epilepsy syndrome, juvenile myoclonic epilepsy (JME) first presents at ages 8–26 years, though typically during teenage years, and accounts for ~10% of all cases of epilepsy. Approximately 30% of those with JME have a familial history of epilepsy.

The characteristic seizure semiology of JME is a bilateral myoclonic seizure often leading to dropping things. This typically occurs in the mornings, leading patients to seek help with a chief complaint of "morning clumsiness" and "tremor during breakfast." The other two main seizure semiologies are dialeptic seizures (loss of awareness) and generalized tonic–clonic seizures. Oftentimes, the first seizure presentation that brings the patients to the attention of a physician is a generalized tonic–clonic seizure. A large proportion of JME patients have significant photosensitivity, ~30%.

The characteristic interictal EEG findings are generalized polyspike and spike-slow wave discharges. Commonly used antiseizure medications are valproic acid, benzodiazepines, levetiracetam, and topiramate. Na-channel blockers like lamotrigine can also be used, especially for generalized tonic–clonic seizures. However, there is a possibility that these could make the myoclonic seizures worse.

In the majority of cases, sustained remission can be achieved; however, anti-seizure medications are often required to be continued because relapse rates are high.

58

• • • • •

Most Malignant of cell type,
Fourth of four, most wild, most hype,
Will brightly glow with gad contrast,
With center dark, and will spread fast.

Hint #1

Look for an area of central necrosis.

Hint #2

Median survival is one year.

Glioblastoma Multiforme

Glioblastoma multiforme (GBM) is the most common primary malignant brain tumor in adults. It is classified as WHO Grade IV amongst primary brain tumors. GBM most commonly affects patients in their 40s–60s with a mean age of 54 years. It is more common in males (1.5:1) and in white individuals (2:1) compared to African Americans. Anatomically, GBM most often arises from the temporal (32%) or frontal lobes (31%). Though GBM is highly locally invasive, it rarely metastasizes outside of the CNS.

The most common symptoms of GBM include headaches and seizures. Focal neurological deficits like weakness, aphasia, and visual field deficits are also commonly observed in patients depending upon the location of the tumor.

Though confirmation requires a biopsy, GBM is often initially diagnosed on a brain MRI, commonly showing hypointensity on T1 sequence with increased T2/FLAIR signal. These are often surrounded by a large area of vasogenic edema, which also appears hyperintense on T2/FLAIR sequence. The T1 post-Gadolinium sequence shows heterogenous enhancement with "central clearing," consistent with a necrotic core. These tumors often have a well-circumscribed lobulated or multilobulated appearance. Rarely, these appear as infiltrating, expansile lesions with vague and ill-defined hyperintensity on T2/FLAIR with minimal edema and no contrast enhancement.

Magnetic resonance spectroscopy (MRS) shows increased choline and decreased N-acetylaspartate in these tumors.

The typical histopathological hallmark of GBM includes microvascular proliferation and necrosis. Both GBM and oligodendrogliomas are classified as diffuse gliomas. If a diffuse glioma has 1p/19q codeletion, it is classified as oligodendroglioma. Those without this mutation are further classified based on other molecular markers, including IDH (isocitrate dehydrogenase), H3 K27, and H3 G34.

For a surgically accessible tumor, maximal surgical resection is the mainstay of the treatment. It is associated with prolonged survival. Many centers use 5-ALA (aminolevulinic acid) for better intraoperative tumor visualization to maximize resection. All patients with GBM must be treated with adjuvant radiation and chemotherapy. For patients with IDH-mutant status with positive MGMT-methylation, the prognosis is better and standard therapy includes temozolomide. It can be used in combination with lomustine. For patients with MGMT-unmethylated tumors, the prognosis is poor and no standard therapy is recommended. These patients are often enrolled in clinical trials.

59

• • • • •

With 3 subtypes, P,C, and A,
Parkinsonism on display,
"Hot Cross" in C, type A will fall,
Dopa will not help type P at all.

Hint #1

Look for decreased metabolism in the cerebellum and striatum on PET scan.

Hint #2

These patients also respond poorly to deep brain stimulation.

Multiple System Atrophy

Neurodegenerative diseases that mimic idiopathic Parkinson disease are often grouped under "Parkinson-plus syndromes." Multiple system atrophy (MSA) is one such disease. It is a synucleinopathy similar to idiopathic Parkinson disease. Based on the predominant symptoms, MSA is divided into three categories.

Multiple system atrophy-Parkinsonian type (MSA-P), formerly known as striatoniagral degeneration, is characterized by parkinsonian features of rigidity, bradykinesia, and a postural tremor, rather than a rest tremor. However, unlike Parkinson disease, symptoms of MSA-P have little to no improvement after treatment with levodopa. Other motor phenomena seen include cortical myoclonus, dystonia, and chorea. Camptocormia and severe anterocollis are more common than in Parkinson disease.

Multiple system atrophy-autonomic type (MSA-A), formally known as Shy-Drager syndrome, has the same Parkinsonian symptoms as those of MSA-P; however, it is differentiated from other MSA subtypes by its symptomatic autonomic dysfunction. The most prominent autonomic sign in MSA-A is often orthostatic hypotension, and many patients experience bowel and bladder dysfunction and impotence. MSA patients often have associated Raynaud phenomenon leading to cold, dusky extremities known as "cold hands sign."

Multiple systems atrophy-cerebellar type (MSA-C), formally known as olivopontocerebellar atrophy mainly has cerebellar signs of progressive gait and limb ataxia, gaze-evoked nystagmus and dysarthria. The pathogenesis of MSA-C is characterized by degeneration of the cerebellum, ventral pons, olives, basal ganglia, and the substantia nigra.

About 15–40% of MSA patients have laryngospasm, leading to stridor, which can be life-threatening. Up to two-thirds of MSA patients also have RBD.

On neuroimaging with MRI, cases of MSA-P can often show decreased signal intensity of the putamen or the "putaminal rim sign" seen as a linear region of hyperintensity surrounding the lateral portion of the putamen on T2 and ADC sequences. Additionally, though not always present, the pontocerebellar tract degeneration of MSA-C can often be seen as a cross-shaped hyperintensity in the pons, called the "hot cross bun sign." A PET scan can also be useful for diagnosis, which will show cerebellar and striatal hypometabolism.

The characteristic finding on histopathology is alpha-synuclein positive glial cytoplasmic inclusions.

These patients respond very poorly to L-Dopa. Treatment is supportive. Recognition of stridor is very important as these patients might require a tracheostomy.

60

• • • • •

Fever, rigid, change is thinking,
High CK, better with drinking,
High blood pressure, high heart rate,
Dopamine blocking drugs create.

Hint #1

A notable lack of clonus.

Hint #2

This condition's name can be confused with a cancer that is metastatic.

Neuroleptic Malignant Syndrome

Neuroleptic malignant syndrome (NMS) is characterized by the triad of hyperthermia, altered mental status, and extrapyramidal symptoms such as rigidity or dyskinesia. NMS is typically associated with the use of dopamine-receptor blocking (DRB) agents such as antipsychotic medications. The signs and symptoms of NMS develop rapidly and most often reach maximum severity within 72 hours of the first onset. The exact pathogenesis of NMS is not well understood.

The hyperthermia of NMS is often accompanied by signs of autonomic dysregulation such as blood pressure lability, tachycardia, and diaphoresis. Elevated CK levels are often seen with the extrapyramidal signs of NMS like rigidity and dyskinesia. And the changes in mentation are usually milder, such as confusion and agitation, rather than stupor or coma.

Development of NMS can occur anytime during the course of DRB treatment, from hours after the first dose to years into continued therapy. Though typical and atypical antipsychotic medications are most commonly associated with the development of NMS, non-neuroleptic medications with anti-dopaminergic activity such as metoclopramide, domperidone, promethazine, levodopa (withdrawal), and amantadine (withdrawal) have also been found to be associated with its development. Given its direct association with drug exposure and fatality in 10–20% of cases depending on the timing of recognition of NMS, it is important to be able to differentiate NMS from serotonin syndrome, malignant hyperthermia, tardive dyskinesia/dystonic storm, acute generalized Parkinsonism, and acute baclofen withdrawal.

NMS is an emergency and is potentially life-threatening. It is critical to recognize this syndrome and stop the offending agent. That is the cornerstone of treatment. The rest of the management is supportive. Medications like benzodiazepines, dantrolene, and bromocriptine can also be used.

61

• • • • •

Headache, mental status change,
Seizure, blood pressure in high range,
Vision loss, some disc swelling,
Improves if down blood pressure bring.

Hint #1

Not always reversible and not always posterior.

Hint #2

Not uncommonly seen in cases of cocaine use and pheochromocytoma.

Posterior Reversible Encephalopathy Syndrome

Posterior reversible encephalopathy syndrome (PRES) is best characterized by a combination of clinico-radioligical signs and symptoms caused by vasogenic brain edema. Patients with PRES most commonly present with a combination of headache, visual disturbance, altered mentation, seizures, and papilledema, in the setting of severe hypertension. Since the edema is mainly located in the posterior cortical regions, visual field deficits and cortical blindness are common presenting symptoms. Simple visual auras could occur as a result of seizure activity involving the occipital lobes.

Though PRES is most commonly found in patients with long-standing hypertension, as well as highly fluctuating severe hypertension as in the cases of pheochromocytoma and cocaine use, a history of elevated blood pressure is not a requirement for diagnosis and is found in only ~75% of cases. Posterior reversible encephalopathy syndrome has also been seen as a complication of pregnancy, particularly eclampsia and HELLP syndrome, as well as a rare complication of chemotherapy, organ transplant, and autoimmune disorders such as systemic lupus. Immunosuppressive medications are being increasingly recognized as a cause for PRES. Common agents include cyclosporine, tacrolimus, and R-CHOP cancer regimen.

The imaging findings of PRES can be striking, with MRI (superior to CT in cases of PRES) often showing bilateral cerebral edema, most commonly prominent in the parietal and occipital lobes. In severe cases, the cerebral edema of PRES can involve deeper brain structures, including the basal ganglia, as well as patchy areas of cerebral ischemia and even hemorrhage.

The management involves blood pressure control and anti-seizure medications for seizures.

62

• • • • •

Post-procedure or nearby,
Infection this pocket will lie,
Can push on nerves from outside in,
Evacuate, culture begin.

Hint #1

Most common bug came from normal skin staphylococcus in spinal, streptococcus if cranial.

Hint #2

Approximately 40% of cases never find a source.

Epidural Abscess

In the CNS, epidural abscesses are usually categorized by location, either cranial or extracranial. Cranial epidural abscesses form outside of the arachnoid and dura mater and are most commonly caused by streptococcal species, then staphylococci, then anaerobic bacteria. Epidural abscesses are also commonly formed at or nearby the area of a surgery. In the case of these nosocomial abscesses, *Pseudomonas* and other species of Gram-negative bacteria are most common.

There are many syndromes associated with cranial epidural abscess formation at or near the skull base, all associated with different cranial nerve involvement. Below is a list of these syndromes starting with the most anteriorly located abscesses.

Foix–Jefferson Syndrome

This abscess located in the cavernous sinus is caused by ethmoid/sphenoid sinusitis (or mucormycosis). It affects CNs III, IV, V-1, V-2, V-3, and VI, producing ophthalmoparesis, eye pain, exophthalmos, and hemi-facial numbness.

Tolosa–Hunt Syndrome

Located on the lateral wall of the cavernous sinus, this cranial epidural abscess is very similar to Foix–Jefferson syndrome; however, it only affects CNs II, IV, V-1, and VI, producing ophthalmoparesis, eye pain, exophthalmos, and facial numbness limited to the forehead (V-1 territory).

Gradenigo Syndrome

Often caused by otitis or mastoiditis and an abscess located at the tip of the petrous bone, Gradenigo syndrome affects CN V and VI, causing diplopia (lateral rectus palsy), severe lateral facial pain, and ear pain.

Vernet Syndrome

Also caused by otitis externa or mastoiditis, though with abscess formation at the jugular foramen at the skull base, this syndrome effects CN IX, X, and XI causing dysphagia, hoarseness, pharyngeal numbness, and weakness of the trapezius muscle.

Collet–Sicard Syndrome

This syndrome is caused by skull base lesions near the jugular foramen, presenting with similar findings to Vernet syndrome but with the addition of CNXII palsy as well. CNXII does not exit via the jugular foramen, but rather via the hypoglossal canal.

Villaret Syndrome

This syndrome is caused by retropharyngeal abscess in the skull base or retroparotid lymphadenitis and affecting CNs IX–XII and the sympathetic chain. It shows the same signs/symptoms as Vernet syndrome plus miosis, tongue weakness, and enophthalmos.

Spinal epidural abscesses (extracranial abscess) are typically divided by location into anterior or posterior abscesses. Posterior spinal abscesses are most often located in the vertical sleeve between the vertebral column and the dura. Typically formed by hematogenous spread, posterior spinal abscesses are much more commonly associated with development at post-traumatic or surgical sites. Anterior spinal abscesses are less likely to form post-procedurally and are most often caused by nearby vertebral body or disk infection. Though symptoms of spinal abscesses often take days to weeks to develop, symptoms that occur over minutes to hours should spark concern for spinal infarction. Native skin staphylococcal species are the most common causal bacteria in spinal epidural abscesses.

Localized back pain is the most common (~75%) symptom of epidural spinal abscess, followed by fever (~50%), and focal neurological deficits (~33%). Bloodwork often shows neutrophilic leukocytosis and elevated CRP and ESR. If lumbar puncture can be performed safely (not near the area of infection), CSF analysis can show elevated WBC, elevated protein, and normal glucose. Neuroimaging of spinal epidural abscesses usually shows extension of the abscess for ≥ 2 adjacent vertebrae and inflammatory involvement/destruction of the surrounding tissues. Contrasted MRI is highly sensitive and often shows focal subarachnoid space enhancement, decreased intervertebral disk space signal, and surrounding bone destruction and edema.

Treatment of these abscesses often requires a combination of antibiotics and surgical exploration with the evacuation of the abscess.

63

• • • • •

Third most common primary,
No periods, sometimes dairy,
Predisposed MEN1,
Both sides outward vision is none.

Hint #1

Men and women present very differently.

Hint #2

Can produce as hypo- and/or hyperactive axis.

Pituitary Adenoma

As the third most common primary brain tumor (~16%), pituitary adenomas are more common in women than in men, and are a known comorbidity of multiple endocrine neoplasia type 1 syndrome. Pituitary adenomas are typically categorized into "secretory," which usually overproduce one or more hormones, or "nonsecretory," which grow and compress adjacent structures.

Nonsecretory pituitary adenomas are the most common type, and with their growth both inside and later outside of the sella they compress structures such as the third ventricle, optic chiasm, hypothalamus, and normal pituitary tissue. The compression of the optic chiasm creates a slowly progressive bitemporal hemianopia and impaired visual acuity, though asymmetric adenomas can compress a single optic nerve, causing unilateral visual impairment. A tumor at the junction of an optic nerve and the optic chiasm can present with the junctional scotoma – ipsilateral central scotoma and contralateral superior temporal scotoma. Rarely, a large pituitary tumor can produce optic atrophy in one eye due to direct compression and papilledema in the other eye due to increased intracranial pressure, a condition known as *Foster Kennedy syndrome*. Compressive nonsecretory pituitary adenomas can compress adjacent healthy anterior pituitary tissue creating hypopituitarism, resulting in hypothyroidism, fatigue, and hypogonadism, while compressions of the posterior pituitary can produce diabetes insipidus. Additionally, larger adenomas can compress the hypothalamus, leading to changes in sleep, mood, and eating habits, while even larger adenomas can compress the third ventricle causing hydrocephalus.

Secretory pituitary adenomas are most commonly prolactinomas (~40%) and commonly cause sexual dysfunction in men and amenorrhea and galactorrhea in women. The second most common type of secretory pituitary adenoma is growth hormone-secreting adenoma, causing gigantism in youth and acromegaly in adults. Though less commonly occurring, adreno-corticotropic hormone-secreting adenomas result in increased cortisol secretion from adrenal glands and cause Cushing disease.

Bloodwork for hormone imbalance is routine and typically consists of prolactin and growth hormone levels, AM cortisol levels, and thyroid function testing. On contrasted MRI, smaller microadenomas (<1 cm) will usually appear hypointense while the adjacent normal gland tissue enhances. Macroadenomas (> 1 cm) will have homogenous enhancement. The treatment of large adenomas often requires surgery.

64

• • • • •

Poor immune, most with type B,
Subacute focal symptoms see,
Increased lymphocytes from back,
High Bar, hot SPECT, and blood will
not lack.

Hint #1

Most commonly of the B-cell variety.

Hint #2

Has a frontal lobe predominance.

Central Nervous System Lymphoma

Approximately 90% of primary and secondary CNS lymphomas are diffuse large B-cell lymphomas, with the minority made up of T-cell lymphomas, Burkitt lymphomas, and low-grade lymphomas. Primary CNS lymphoma is highly associated with HIV, and is the second most common cause of brain mass lesion (CNS toxoplasmosis is first) in patients with coexisting late-stage HIV and CD4 + T-lymphocyte count of <50 cells/μL. Though CNS lymphoma is more common in men than in women with an average age of diagnosis of ~55 years, patients with coexisting AIDS are usually diagnosed at a much younger age of ~35 years. The Epstein–Barr virus (EBV) is found in ~99% of patients with AIDS-related primary CNS lymphoma, while found in ~90% of the general population. Patients with EBV + primary CNS lymphoma have a poorer prognosis than EBV patients as the EBV genome has been found to express anti-apoptotic genes in its genome, leading to malignant transformation of cancer cells.

The clinical presentation of primary CNS lymphoma is usually a subacute progression of headache, focal neurological deficits, encephalopathy, and eventually seizures, usually in the absence of fever or other systemic symptoms. Cerebral spinal fluid analysis usually shows a lymphocyte-predominant pleocytosis with normal glucose but slightly elevated protein concentration. Obtaining an EBV PCR is very important, though it neither confirms nor excludes the presence or absence, respectively, of primary CNS lymphoma. Cytology and flow cytometry of collected CSF cells can also help with lymphoma subtyping.

Most commonly seen as an enhancing single isolated lesion, or less often as multiple enhancing lesions on contrasted MRI or CT, primary CNS lymphoma has a predominance for the periventricular area and the frontal lobes. In contrast to toxoplasmosis, lesions are not ring-enhancing, but rather heterogeneously enhancing, and can cross the midline through the corpus collosum. Another characteristic feature is that primary CNS lymphoma shows diffusion restriction. Another way to differentiate primary CNS lymphoma from toxoplasmosis is by thallium SPECT imaging, which will show increased thallium uptake, also known as "hot." Additionally, perfusion-weighted imaging usually shows increased regional blood flow in the area of the lesion, differentiating it from CNS toxoplasmosis, which shows areas of decreased blood flow. Definitive diagnosis comes with brain biopsy.

Once the biopsy has been obtained, dexamethasone can be used for symptomatic management. The cornerstone of chemotherapy is methotrexate, in combination with rituximab.

65

· · · · ·

Seizures with changes in tone,
Rarely controlled with meds alone,
In kids you'll see slow spike and wave,
Delays in how they will behave.

Hint #1

Most commonly presents with tonic seizures.

Hint #2

Usually diagnosed in patients between 3–5 years old.

Lennox–Gastaut Syndrome

Lennox–Gastaut syndrome (LGS) is a severe developmental epileptic encephalopathy, characterized by refractory epilepsy, developmental delay, and severe intellectual disability. The onset is usually before the age of 8 years. Various seizure semiologies are observed in LGS patients, including tonic, atonic, myoclonic, and dialeptic seizures. The most common seizure semiology is tonic seizure.

Lennox–Gastaut syndrome can be caused by a variety of etiologies including hypoxic-ischemic insults, malformations of cortical development, neurocutaneous syndromes such as tuberous sclerosis, and CNS infections such as meningitis and encephalitis. About one-fourth of LGS patients has a preceding history of epileptic spasms and West syndrome.

The most characteristic interictal EEG finding is a generalized slow spike and wave discharge (<2.5 Hz). Another characteristic finding is generalized paroxysmal fast activity. Tonic seizures are associated with an electrodecrement with or without associated fast activity.

Treatment options include medications such as valproate, clobazam, topiramate, cannabidiol, and fenfluramine. Atonic seizures, in particular, respond very well to corpus callosotomy.

66

• • • • •

Granulomas, nerves to face,
Chest X ray, CSF ACE,
Will see on contrast MRI,
Biopsy and should steroids try.

Hint #1

Commonly produces upper and lower facial droop.

Hint #2

Can also produce meningeal disease.

Neurosarcoidosis

Though sarcoidosis commonly involves the nervous system sub-clinically (~50% found postmortem), clinically evident neurological disease is only present in ~10% of patients with sarcoidosis. Once sarcoidosis involves the nervous system, the so-called neurosarcoidosis can involve any part of the neuroaxis and produce a spectrum of clinical manifestations including cranial neuropathies, intra- and extra-axial granulomatous disease, meningeal disease, and cerebral white matter disease.

The most common presenting signs of neurosarcoidosis are cranial neuropathies, and the most common cranial nerve affected is CN 7, causing weakness of the upper and lower face, which can present bilaterally. Hearing and balance dysfunction is also a common presenting symptom from the involvement of CN 8. Studies show large variation in the frequency of involvement of other CNs; however, involvement of CN 1-4 and 6 has also been reported and is associated with granulomatous compression or invasion of the CNs in the orbit.

Neurosarcoidosis infrequently presents as meningitis that can in-turn cause multiple cranial neuropathies and/or hydrocephalus. This form of meningitis often affects the dura more than the arachnoid, hence called pachymeningitis. The granulomatous disease of the spinal cord often causes myelopathic symptoms, and the involvement of the hypothalamus in cerebral disease often causes significant endocrinopathies. Distal, symmetrical polyneuropathies and mononeuropathy multiplex can be seen in cases where the peripheral nervous system is involved.

In general, but more commonly associated with meningeal disease, CSF analysis will show a mononuclear pleocytosis with high protein concentration and low to normal CSF glucose. Elevated levels of angiotensin-converting enzyme (ACE) in the serum and CSF can be helpful; however, it lacks sensitivity.

Nervous tissue biopsy showing noncaseating granuloma is required for definitive diagnosis, though in the case of known systemic sarcoidosis, the diagnosis can be presumed with corroborating CSF analysis, clinical presentation, and neuroimaging findings. It should be noted however that the possibility of other diagnoses should be eliminated if the patient has been on immunosuppressive therapy.

Steroids form the cornerstone of treatment for both acute and chronic diseases. For chronic use, steroid-sparing agents like mycophenolate, azathioprine, cyclophosphamide, and methotrexate can be used as well.

67

• • • • •

Ophthalmoplegia, reflex decline,
And trouble walking in a line,
Some have eye pain, but can see,
And have anti-GQ1B.

Hint #1

Hint #1

A small percentage of Guillain–Barré syndrome.

Hint #2

Not typically associated with profound limb weakness.

Miller Fisher Syndrome

Miller Fisher syndrome (MFS) is a variant of Guillain–Barré syndrome (GBS), which is characterized by the clinical triad of ophthalmoplegia, areflexia, and ataxia. Overall, it constitutes ~5–10% of all GBS cases.

This clinical triad was first described in 1932 by English neurologist James Collier and later by Canadian neurologist Charles Miller Fisher in 1965.

Miller Fisher syndrome is characterized by the presence of anti-GQ1b antibodies. Overall, there are three main anti-GQ1b variants – MFS, Bickerstaff brainstem encephalitis, and pharyngeal-cervical–brachial (PCB) variant.

Like typical GBS, CSF analysis in the case of MFS will typically show albuminocytologic dissociation though 10% of cases have no abnormalities in CSF, as changes in CSF concentrations are most pronounced 2–4 weeks after symptom onset. Conduction studies may show slowing of sensory nerve conduction. If the patients develop clinical weakness, then the nerve conduction studies might demonstrate findings similar to AIDP.

The management is similar to AIDP. Patients must be admitted to hospital with telemetry monitoring. Acute treatment options include IVIG and plasma exchange.

68

• • • • •

Both hemispheres involved, you'll see,
Stiffness, shaking, eyes open be,
Lactate/creatine kinase high,
Give Benzos quick, turn to side lie.

Hint #1

Finding the right answer is nothing to ictal cry about.

Hint #2

Do not bite your tongue. Just say what you are thinking.

Generalized Tonic–Clonic Seizure

A generalized tonic-clonic (GTC) seizure is characterized by whole body stiffening (tonic phase), followed by whole body jerking or twitching movements (clonic phase). In some cases, there is a clonic phase preceding the tonic phase, thus leading to a clonic-tonic-clonic sequence.

During the tonic phase, the arms can be in an extended posture (decerebrate) with the wrists and metacarpophalangeal joints being hyper-flexed. The index fingers are usually extended to interphalangeal joints, while the rest of the fingers are flexed, as if the index fingers are pointing downward. In some cases, the arms are held in a flexed posture (decorticate). During the tonic phase, the neck is extended with eyes rolled upward. The tonic phase is often associated with a loud scream at the onset known as the *ictal cry*. This sign is very specific for the episode to be of epileptic origin.

The tonic phase is then followed by a jittery phase, which is characterized by fast irregular jerky movements superimposed on underlying tonic contraction. The jittery phase is then followed by the clonic phase. Clonic contractions are essentially short tetanic contractions, interrupted by silent periods. The frequency of the clonic contractions decreases as the seizure progresses. This is mainly because of progressive prolongation of the silent periods.

GTC seizures can be primary (as seen in generalized epilepsies) or secondary (as seen in focal epilepsies). The secondarily generalized tonic-clonic seizures are usually asynchronous between the two sides.

Most GTC seizures stop within 2–3 minutes. Prolonged and more frequent GTC seizures are associated with increased risk of SUDEP. The EEG after a GTC seizure can show generalized suppression. This phase is considered to be a marker of cerebral hypoxia. It is often clinically associated with postictal tonic posturing. Postictal EEG suppression and postictal central apnea are potential biomarkers for SUDEP.

69

• • • • •

Stabbing pain, up to hundreds per day,
In and around one eye,
With tears and lacrimation,
On AED's rely.

Hint #1

Attacks last seconds to minutes.

Hint #2

Involves injection but no needle.

Short-Lasting Unilateral Neuralgiform Attacks with Conjunctival Injection and Tearing Syndrome (SUNCT)

Also known by its abbreviation SUNCT, short-lasting unilateral neuralgiform attacks with conjunctival injection and tearing syndrome is the rarest type of the trigeminal autonomic cephalgias. Those with SUNCT suffer multiple days of painful "attacks" characterized by a sharp stabbing or pulsatile pain located in or around one eye or temporal area. Attacks occur up to 200 times per day, lasting only 5 seconds to 4 minutes each, and are accompanied by autonomic symptoms, such as lacrimation and/or conjunctival injection that occurs ipsilateral to the facial pain. Patients with SUNCT also report that these attacks can often be triggered by touching the area affected by the attack or even moving their head. Between attacks, most patients report no pain, though some report a lingering dull painful sensation.

The diagnosis is clinical and is supported by lack of response to indomethacin. The acute attacks are treated by IV lidocaine infusion. Preventive options include lamotrigine, gabapentin, and topiramate. Lamotrigine is likely the most effective preventive medication for SUNCT.

70

● ● ● ● ●

A headache both diffuse and dull,
And product of a leak,
Standing induced, resolves supine,
A patch is what you seek.

Hint #1

Do not know the answer? Do not worry. There is low pressure.

Hint #2

Most commonly iatrogenically caused.

Intracranial Hypotension Headache

Also called "low-pressure headaches," intracranial hypotension headaches are most commonly caused by low CSF pressure due to a CSF leak through a dural leak, like after lumbar puncture. These leaks can also result from spine surgeries, erosion of the sinuses and/or the skull, and even vigorous exercise, while low CSF volume without a causal leak can occur due to severe dehydration and uremia.

Those with an intracranial hypotension headache usually complain of a holocephalic, dull, or throbbing type pain that is worse with standing or sitting up from a lying position, and better lying flat. In cases of chronic low-pressure headache, these patients can begin showing meningeal and migrainous signs such as nuchal rigidity, nausea and vomiting, photophobia, and tinnitus.

For patients with no obvious cause, an MRI of the brain with and without Gad is required to detect a potential leak. Other modalities to detect a leak include MR myelography without Gad or radioisotope cisternography.

Treatment options include bedrest and caffeine intake. For patients with severe symptoms or refractory symptoms, an epidural blood patch can be used.

71

• • • • •

Oft times with trauma history,
EEG to diagnose,
Normal waves but you can see,
Eyes closed, pedaling, no benzos.

Hint #1

Make your conversion over to the right answer.

Hint #2

Look for a history of abuse.

Psychogenic Nonepileptic Seizures

Also called psychogenic seizures, nonepileptic seizures or pseudo-seizures, functional seizures, psychogenic nonepileptic seizures (PNES) are characterized by episodes of seizure-like activity without true epileptiform activity detected on EEG. The pathophysiology of these episodes is poorly understood, though an active area of research. There is a higher prevalence of PNES in women as well as in those with a history of psychological, physical, or sexual trauma or abuse.

Signs and symptoms of PNES can be very similar to those found in epileptic seizures. In general, characteristics more consistent with PNES than typical epileptic seizures are a recently preceding emotional disturbance, the appearance of irregularly "throwing" limbs around rather than stereotyped rhythmic jerking, episodes lasting for many minutes, a fluctuating seizure course, and no postictal confusion or fatigue. The diagnosis of PNES can be very difficult as some studies show that up to 50% of those with PNES also have epileptic seizures. Continuous video EEG monitoring is required to diagnose PNES.

It is critical to be as certain of the diagnosis as possible. It is also very important to establish if the patient has coexisting epilepsy because that would warrant treatment with anti-seizure medications. Frontal lobe epilepsy can often present with hypermotor seizures, which are characterized by complex bicycling or pedaling movements. Rarely, patients can jump out of the bed and run around. Patients with frontal lobe epilepsy often get misdiagnosed with non-epileptic seizures.

The treatment of these patients is difficult and requires a multi-disciplinary approach with psychiatrists and psychologists. Psychotherapy is very important. Options include cognitive behavioral therapy (CBT), mindfulness-based therapy, and psychodynamic interpersonal therapy. Some factors that predict poor prognosis include longer duration of symptoms, older age of onset, rejection of the diagnosis, and severe underlying psychiatric disorder.

72

• • • • •

Hand moves at rest, and shuffled feet,
With neurotransmitter deplete,
Not a "plus," eyes move just fine,
No hot cross bun or avian sign.

Hint #1

Treat by replacing and/or implanting.

Hint #2

Originally the "shaking palsy."

Parkinson Disease

First described by English surgeon and apothecary Dr. James Parkinson in 1817, the disease now known as Parkinson disease (PD) was first described in a 66-page treatise entitled *An Essay on the Shaking Palsy*, a disease he first names "Paralysis Agitans." PD is a neurodegenerative disease, characterized by abnormal deposition of alpha-synculein. Histopathologically, the brain tissue of those with PD demonstrates eosinophilic cytoplasmic inclusions called *Lewy bodies*. The Braak hypothesis suggests that the synucleinopathy in idiopathic PD follows a specific pattern with initial deposition seen in dorsal motor nucleus of the vagus that spreads through the brain in a prion-like fashion. The involvement of dopaminergic neurons in the substantia nigra pars compacta leads to the motor signs of idiopathic PD.

Multiple gene mutations have been linked to the development of PD. Some of the well-established monogenic causes of PD include mutations in SNCA, LRRK2, PRKN, PINK1, and DJ-1 genes. The most common of these is the LRRK2 gene mutation. Some other gene mutations are known to increase the risk of, rather than cause, PD. One of these is the GBA1 mutation, which causes Gaucher disease.

Signs of PD begin on average in patients' 50s, and they include bradykinesia, resting tremor, impaired postural reflexes, rigidity, and altered gait. Symptoms progress slowly, with resting tremor and rigidity typically starting unilaterally. By the time signs are clinically evident, the patient has already lost ~60% of their dopaminergic neurons and ~80% of the dopamine in their nigrostriatal pathway.

The majority of patients first seek care because of a resting tremor, which is typically 4–5 Hz in frequency, primarily in one upper extremity, most prominent in the hand and wrist, and lessens with action. The resting tremor of PD often extends to the ipsilateral leg, and then slowly generalizes to the contralateral limbs, often also progressing to affect the trunk, lips, jaw, and tongue. The bradykinesia of PD is evident with impairment of rapid and repetitive fine motor movements, tested clinically with finger and toe tapping. Additionally, bradykinesia is seen in the impaired gait of these patients and characterized by stooped posture, reduced arm swing, shuffled stepping, and freezing episodes of immobility. Lastly, this bradykinesia can be evidenced by decreased facial expression (hypomimia), quiet voice (hypophonia), and decreased blink rate. The limb rigidity of PD often becomes evident after the tremor and bradykinesia if present. Most prominent in the limbs, patients with PD develop an increased sustained resistance to passive movements. This can also be evidenced by "cogwheeling" of the limb, in which the effects of rigidity and tremor can both be felt by the examiner as a ratchet-like stop and start motion during passive range of motion.

The "freezing" of gait in PD, so called motor blocks freezing episodes most often occur during specific times and scenarios such as when attempting to initiate stepping, while turning, crossing, or arriving at some sort of visual but not obstructive boundary such as across a line, through a doorway, or arriving at a chair. Another gait characteristic of PD is festination, during which the patient begins to take progressively faster but shorter steps. Gait in PD is also affected by impaired postural reflexes. This is evident clinically when the patient has difficulty maintaining balance or will retropulse when the clinician slightly pulls the patient from behind. Freezing, festination, and loss of postural reflexes are typically later signs in PD.

Unlike Dr. Parkinson's original description, PD can have profound non-motor symptoms that can occur years before motor signs/symptoms. These included mood (anxiety, depression), cognitive (bradyphrenia and eventual dementia), behavioral (changes in personality and attention), autonomic (constipation, impotence, urinary retention), sensory (limb pain/paresthesia), and even sleep (REM sleep behavior disorder) symptoms.

No serum or CSF tests can diagnose PD, but rather help eliminate mimicking conditions, and diagnosis relies on a precise clinical history and neuroimaging. MRI is typically unremarkable in PD. Single-photon emission computed tomography (SPECT) uses the radiopharmaceutical ^{123}I-ioflupane and helps to visualize the basal ganglia dopamine transporters. This study is also known as a DaTscan. In the appropriate clinic picture, and with a DaTscan showing decreased marker uptake, PD-related tremor can be distinguished from essential tremor, though cannot be differentiated from other types of so-called Parkinson-plus disorders. Positron emission tomography scan with the radioactive L-DOPA analog F-fluorodopa can also help establish a diagnosis of PD. This scan will show a decreased uptake of fluorodopa in the basal ganglia in cases of PD. Though neuroimaging can be helpful, the diagnosis of PD can be made by clinical history and exam alone.

The treatment of PD is mainly symptomatic. L-Dopa is the key treatment option available that helps the symptoms of tremor and bradykinesia the most. In addition, dopamine agonists like ropinirole or pramipexole are often used in younger patients with high risk of dyskinesias. For very mild disease, MAO-B inhibitors like rasagiline are a good option. For tremor-predominant PD, anticholinergics like trihexylphenidyl and amantadine are good options. Deep brain stimulation has revolutionized the treatment of PD. Generally speaking, patients who are responsive to L-Dopa are good candidates for DBS.

73

• • • • •

Continuous but worse at times,
Head pain all on one side,
With tears, red eyes, and runny nose,
Indomethacin provide.

Hint #1

Unlike the answer, the riddle is a pain in the neck.

Hint #2

Needle-like pain.

Hemicrania Continua

Also one of the four trigeminal autonomic cephalgias, hemicrania continua (HC) is known for being indomethacin-responsive (the other being chronic paroxysmal hemicrania). The signs and symptoms of HC are notably completely unilateral and consist of moderate to severe continuous side-lock headache without painless periods, lasting for more than three months. This prolonged headache period can fluctuate in intensity and during exacerbations must also occur with at least one sign of autonomic involvement ipsilateral to the headache such as conjunctival injection, lacrimation, nasal congestion, rhinorrhea, miosis, or ptosis. Patients with HC also commonly complain of a sharp, needle-like orbital and temporal pain. Though neuroimaging is relatively unremarkable in most cases of headache, a small study in 2004 did show that PET scans of those with HC did show activation of the ipsilateral rostral pons and contralateral posterior hypothalamus.

Patients with HC often respond well to 75–150 mg/day of indomethacin, though symptoms can return, often requiring life-long prophylactic dosing.

74

•••••

With trauma or adjustment comes,
Fast headache and neck pain,
Horner knows, CTA shows,
Two lumens, deprived brain.

Hint #1

Treat by dissolving or stabilizing.

Hint #2

Look out for ptosis and miosis.

Carotid or Vertebral Dissection

Carotid dissections and vertebral dissections cause ~20% of strokes in patients <45 years old and can be caused by direct trauma to or round the neck, whiplash injury, violent coughing, strenuous events like exercise or childbirth, or occur spontaneously. Arterial dissections are also more common in patients with connective tissue disease such as Marfan, Loeys–Deitz, and Ehlers–Danlos syndromes; osteogenesis imperfecta; fibromuscular dysplasia; and α_1-antitrypsin deficiency. Carotid dissections are much more common than vertebral dissections, comprising ~70–80% of all cervicocerebral arterial dissections, and vertebral dissections comprising ~15%.

During arterial dissection, a tear in the wall leads to a collection of blood between the walls of the artery, ultimately producing an intramural hematoma. The hematoma can produce luminal narrowing and can expand and rupture into the true lumen of the artery. Both of these scenarios predispose the patient to a high likelihood of local thrombus formation and/or embolism.

Signs and symptoms of a carotid dissection or vertebral dissections typically include sudden ipsilateral headache and neck pain around the area of dissection. These are often described to be sharp and can involve the ipsilateral jaw/face. Headaches can be severe and are sometimes considered "thunderclap"-type headaches. Horner syndrome can occur in patients with cervical carotid artery dissection because of local swelling of the artery and compression of the surrounding sympathetic plexus. A so-called painful Horner syndrome may be the only presenting symptom. Additionally, patients may complain of pulsatile tinnitus.

Emergent vessel imaging such as the CTA angiogram is often the first investigation. If the intraluminal thrombus causes significant narrowing, then the CTA will simply show that. Sometimes, it shows the false lumen. MRI T1 with fat suppression is the best study to visualize the intramural thrombus.

Secondary stroke prevention in extracranial vascular dissection warrants either antiplatelet therapy or anticoagulant therapy. There is no clear consensus on this. For intracranial vascular dissection, most experts recommend antiplatelet therapy because of a higher risk of bleeding.

75

• • • • •

A variant of otherwise,
A weakness of ascension,
Full sensory and jejuni,
Anti-GM1 retention.

Acute Motor Axonal Neuropathy

A variant of GBS, acute motor axonal neuropathy (AMAN) is estimated to comprise ~5–10% of GBS cases. AMAN and its similar subtype acute motor and sensory neuropathy (AMSAN) cause primary axonal destruction with little to no demyelination. This is unlike the most popular type of GBS, AIDP, in which primary destruction to the peripheral nerve is demyelination. The pathogenesis is thought to be like that of AIDP with a postinfectious humoral antibody-mediated injury to the peripheral nerves.

Weakness in AMAN is typically more rapid than that of AIDP, as flaccid paralysis develops over a week, with atrophy, which is evident earlier in the clinical course, and areflexia. Weakness is bilateral, symmetrical, and affecting the legs more than the arms. Separating it from all other subtypes of GBS, those with AMAN have no sensory disturbance. Respiratory failure is more common in AMAN than in other subtypes.

Compared to AIDP, a higher percentage than with AMAN (~75%) test seropositive for *Campylobacter jejuni*. AMAN also has a higher likelihood of antibodies against gangliosides GM1, GD1a, and GD1b. Electromyography will show reduced motor amplitudes with normal sensory studies. Cerebrospinal fluid analysis often demonstrates elevated protein after two weeks, and it is seen to be most prominent 4–6 weeks after symptom onset. CSF pleocytosis is variable but is typically either absent or small and lymphocytic.

Treatment for all forms of GBS is similar. Patients must be admitted to hospital with telemetry monitoring and frequent respiratory checks. Declining respiratory function would warrant an ICU transfer and noninvasive or invasive ventilation. IVIG and plasma exchange are often used in the acute setting. Compared to patients with AIDP, the recovery in AMAN is much slower and the overall prognosis is poorer because of axonal damage. Nerve conduction studies could help indicate the prognosis. If the CMAP amplitudes are less than 20% of normal with fibrillation potentials and an overall axonal pattern, the prognosis will be poorer compared to a nerve conduction study showing mainly demyelination.

76

• • • • •

A gradual and slow weakness,
Older folks with reflex bleakness,
Demyelination, asensory,
Treat with immunotherapy.

Hint #1

Like GBS, but slower.

Hint #2

More common in those >50.

Chronic Inflammatory Demyelinating Polyradiculoneuropathy

Chronic inflammatory demyelinating polyradiculoneuropathy (CIDP) is a slow, progressive, sensorimotor disease thought to have both a cell-mediated and humoral immune pathogenesis.

Patients typically present with progressive motor and sensory symptoms over months and years, though most present with a primary complaint of weakness. Typical CIDP presents with a symmetric bilateral sensorimotor polyneuropathy with diminished reflexes. Weakness is often much greater than the extent of sensory loss. The difference from any other toxic/metabolic neuropathy is that the pattern of weakness and sensory loss is not length-dependent.

There are many variants of CIDP, such as pure motor and pure sensory forms. Multifocal CIDP, aka Lewis–Sumner syndrome (MADSAM – multifocal-acquired demyelinating sensory and motor neuropathy) presents an asymmetric form of neuropathy, which mimics mononeuropathy multiplex. A very peculiar variant of CIDP that presents with a symmetric length-dependent sensory neuropathy is called DADS (distal-acquired demyelinating symmetric neuropathy). Often difficult to recognize clinically because of its similarities to many other length-dependent neuropathies, it can have additional clinical features such as tremor and cramps. As opposed to typical CIDP, DADS is much more likely to be associated with a monoclonal gammopathy. If positive, ~50% of those patients will have anti-MAG (myelin-associated glycoprotein) antibodies. This is now considered to be a completely different entity than CIDP. Another peculiar variant of CIDP produces a profound sensory ataxia with tremor in younger patients. This variant is associated with antibodies against neurofascin (NF)-155.

Bloodwork and neuroimaging of these patients are typically normal. Analysis of CSF, like GBS, often shows an elevated protein level in the absence of pleocytosis or other irregularity. In these patients, demyelination is often evident on NCS, showing decreased conduction velocities, conduction blocks, prolonged motor latencies, and F waves (atypical late responses). In advanced cases, the secondary axonal loss can be severe enough to prevent detection of demyelination on NCS. In these cases, neuromuscular ultrasound has revolutionized the diagnosis of CIDP. Ultrasound can detect severely enlarged nerve diameters typical of CIDP and can easily distinguish it from other causes of neuropathy.

The treatment of CIDP includes steroids and chronic IVIG. Other options include rituximab, methotrexate, azathioprine, and cyclophosphamide. Rituximab may be effective in anti-MAG neuropathy.

77

• • • • •

Presenting in the youthful most,
After descending rash, years post,
Clonic jerks, mentation blight,
And lesions in subcortical white.

Hint #1

One of many reasons why vaccines are great.

Hint #2

Adult-onset form can occur at around 20 years of age.

Subacute Sclerosing Panencephalitis

Subacute sclerosing panencephalitis (SSPE) is a neurodegenerative disease affecting the CNS, occurring primarily in children aged 7–11, and proving 100% fatal despite treatment. Though the exact pathogenesis of SSPE is not understood, it is generally accepted that SSPE is caused by the persistent, dormant, infection with a genetically variant form of the measles virus. Understandably, SSPE occurs almost entirely in areas with low rates of measles vaccination such as parts of Africa and Asia. Historically only three to five cases occur in the USA yearly; however, this incidence increased three-fold in 2019, a change thought to be linked with the drop in US vaccination rates.

The clinical course of SSPE is highly variable; it is generally divided temporally into four stages. Initial signs of SSPE (stage 1) are progressive cognitive, behavioral, and personality changes such as worsening school performance, irritability, social withdrawal, lethargy, and language regression. Stage 2 of SSPE is primarily characterized by the onset of progressive motor dysfunction such as dyskinesias, dystonia, rigidity, and seizures. There is also a marked decline in mentation in stage 2, often to the point of clinical dementia. Progression to stage 3 is marked by worsening extrapyramidal symptoms such as rigidity and dystonias, as well as progressively worsening seizures. Patients in stage 3 often become bed-bound, incontinent of urine and stool, and fully reliant on others for ADLs. In the final stage of SSPE, stage 4, these patients become akinetic, mute, and enter a vegetative state with death occurring either in stage 3 or 4, within three years of the first symptom onset.

In some cases, visual impairment, mainly focal necrotizing macular retinitis, can precede the clinical onset of SSPE by one to two years. Also, a rarer adult form of SSPE does exist, with an average age of onset being 20. And though the clinical course is similar, this form is more often preceded by visual impairment.

In patients with SSPE, CSF analysis will show albuminocytologic dissociation (elevated protein without pleocytosis), elevated IgG synthesis rates and levels, and positive oligoclonal banding. More specific to SSPE, CSF measles IgG titer >1:4, serum measles IgG titers >1:256, or < 1:200 CSF-to-serum ratio is indicative of a confirmed diagnosis. The sensitivity and specificity of CSF measles RNA PCR is still being investigated.

The EEG findings over the course of SSPE vary widely from those of the early stages showing generalized slowing, then progressing to generalized periodic activity of 2–3-second high-voltage polyphasic delta waves (Raedmecker complex) coinciding with the patient's myoclonic jerks, interrupted by 4–8-second long intervals. Magnetic resonance imaging will show T2 increased signal, primarily in the subcortical white matter, with occipitoparietal predominance in the earlier stages. As SSPE progresses, lesions spread to gray matter, with sparing of the U-fibers.

78

• • • • •

Most common in immune suppressed,
Ubiquitous virus possessed,
Dementia, focal deficits,
White matter and U fiber hits.

Hint #1

Do not know, ask James Cunningham.

Hint #2

Check CSF because serum will almost always be positive.

Progressive Multifocal Leukoencephalopathy

Progressive multifocal leukoencephalopathy (PML) is a fatal neurodegenerative disease characterized by subacute CNS demyelination caused by the reactivation of the dormant human polyomavirus, JC virus (named after James Cunningham, the patient from whom the virus was first isolated). JC virus is considered ubiquitous, with ~70% of healthy individuals possessing JC virus antibodies; these antibodies are thought to remain dormant in the bone marrow or kidneys and get activated at the time of immunosuppression. Though only 1–4% of patients with HIV have PML, usually presenting with CD4 counts below 200 cells/μL, ~80% of those with PML also have HIV. Additionally, those on immunosuppressive therapy, or with hematological malignancies or autoimmune diseases are at a higher risk of developing PML.

Given the multifocality of the demyelinating CNS lesions, there is significant variation in the clinical presentation of PML. In general, patients present with subacute signs and symptoms including cognitive impairment hemiparesis, visual disturbance, ataxia, and sensory loss. Seizure can be present, but is uncommon. Cranial and peripheral nerves remain unaffected and demyelination of the spinal cord is rare. Though routine CSF labs are typically unremarkable, CSF PCR and JC virus DNA are both sensitive (~70–90%) and specific (>90%). Given the ubiquity of JC virus in the general population, serum JC virus PCR and antibody studies are typically unhelpful and generally positive.

An MRI scan most commonly shows multifocal T2/FLAIR hyperintense lesions (though occasionally lesions are found solitary if early in the disease process) with a supratentorial predominance. Brainstem and cerebellar lesions can however be present. Multifocal areas of demyelination seen on imaging begin to involve U-fibers and lesions often appear to coalesce as the disease progresses. Though both hyper and hypometabolic lesions can be seen in FTD-PET scans, these lesions appear very similar to those found in primary CNS lymphoma. Ultimately, the definitive diagnosis is made with brain biopsy.

For patients with HIV, antiretroviral therapy is the key treatment option. Rarely, the initiation of antiretroviral therapy can induce PML-IRIS (immune reconstitution syndrome), which requires steroids. For patients who are immunocompromised because of some other reason, if there is an offending medication like natalizumab, it must be immediately stopped. Specifically for patients with natalizumab medication, plasma exchange is recommended as well.

79

• • • • •

Limb-gait atax the young within,
No reflex or Frataxin,
And GAA shows expansion,
Diabetes, heart issues in.

Hint #1

Most eventually die from heart failure.

Hint #2

Runs in families.

Friedreich Ataxia

Hereditary ataxias are classified based on their inheritance. Amongst autosomal recessive ataxias, Friedreich ataxia (FA) is the most common. Most FA cases are caused by loss-of-function mutations in the frataxin gene on chromosome 9q13. This mutation is characterized by GAA trinucleotide repeat expansion in the noncoding first intron of the frataxin gene, resulting in its silencing and deficiency.

Symptom onset of FA is typically between 2 and 25 years of age and usually begins as a slowly progressive cerebellar limb and gait ataxia. The earlier the age of onset, the more rapid is disease progression. Onset at an earlier age is associated with a higher number of GAA repeats.

The clinical syndrome is characterized by a combination of slowly progressive ataxia, diabetes mellitus, and cardiomyopathy. In addition to the ataxia, other critical neurological findings include a peripheral sensory neuropathy with dorsal column dysfunction and absent reflexes. Skeletal abnormalities like kyphoscoliosis are also very common.

Up to 85% of patients develop hypertrophic cardiomyopathy by early adulthood. It is critical to identify this because arrhythmias and heart failure are very common causes of death in FA patients.

There is no cure for this disease. Management is supportive only.

80

• • • • •

Postflu-like, and then will spread,
To face weakness, inflamed in head,
Neuropathy, in those tick bait,
Ceftriaxone if caught late.

Disseminated Lyme Disease (neuroborreliosis)

Lyme disease is a tick-borne illness caused by the flagellated spirochete *Borrelia burgdorferi*. Clinical presentation often starts with flu-like symptoms that progress to a wide variety of serious neurological conditions known as disseminated Lyme disease, or neuroborreliosis, if untreated. In the United States of America, Lyme disease infections predominantly take place in the northeastern (Pennsylvania, New York, New Jersey, Maine) and northern midwest states (Wisconsin, Minnesota).

The history of the name Lyme disease and its causal spirochete is particularly interesting. In the early 1970s, a group of people in a small rural town in Connecticut began getting ill with severe fatigue, swollen joints, and headache. Two determined mothers of sick children began taking notes and investigating these cases, eventually contacting scientists. Their persistence paid off and by the mid-1970s the group of symptoms were formally recognized as a syndrome, despite not knowing the cause. This syndrome was then named after this community, Lyme disease, hence the capital "L." Later, in 1981, researcher William Bergdorfer and his colleagues discovered spirochetes and were able to trace a specific species back to the deer ticks of Lyme Connecticut. After his findings were published in 1982, the scientific community named the discovered spirochete species after him, *B. burgdorferi*.

The transmission of *B. burgdorferi* to humans begins when the larvae of the blacklegged tick (*Ixodes scapulari*), also known as the deer tick, attach to an already infected host, which is usually a forest rodent such as the white-footed mouse or deer mouse. These tick larvae become infected with *B. burgdorferi* during their blood meal on the rodent, and eventually mature into nymphs and fall off. These infected nymphs then mature into adult ticks and infect humans during a blood meal, or mate on the hides of deer, eventually laying their eggs back on the ground, starting the cycle over.

The first sign of early infection (stage 1) is usually a > 5 cm, red targetoid lesion, known as *erythema migrans*, appearing at the location of the tick bite. Rash appearance varies widely and may appear homogenous or have a central red area rather than central clearing. This rash appears in ~75% of infected patients and can appear anytime from three days to one month after the infecting tick bite. The rash is then typically followed shortly after by a flu-like illness that signifies the beginning of the next stage.

Neurological symptoms begin early in the disseminated infection (stage 2), which most often occurs 2–4 weeks after first inoculation. This stage begins with symptoms of significant fatigue, myalgia, headache, and neck stiffness. Arthralgias, most commonly the knee, commonly occur one-month postinoculation, and are often followed by more serious conditions such as Lyme-carditis, which can cause heart block. These patients also often develop neurological manifestations of neuroborreliosis such as meningeal signs and cranial nerve palsies (~50%), which most commonly affect the facial nerve and can be bilateral.

Stage 3 of the infections has primarily neurological manifestations, consisting of radicular pain, encephalitis, myelitis, and an axonal peripheral neuropathy, all of which usually occur three months after inoculation.

The diagnostic workup for Lyme disease can be difficult as both CSF and serum Lyme serology can take weeks to months to obtain the results, and spirochetes are very difficult to culture. Monocytic and lymphocytic pleocytoses are often present, but often only occur in combination with meningeal signs. Elevated CSF protein is common, CSF antibodies are only found in ~50% of cases, and CSF PCR is only positive in ~50% of those with meningitis. Given the insensitivity of direct forms of testing (such as PCR), the gold standard is a 2-tier approach using indirect forms of anti-borrelia antibody testing such as ELISA, then confirming the diagnosis using Western immunoblot testing. It should be noted, however, that indirect testing has been shown to have crossreactivity to related bacteria species, and some studies have reported the Western blot false-positive rate to be more than 50%.

81

• • • • •

Eyelids spasm on both sides,
In mainly women it resides,
Tongue/throat movements, forced open/close,
Treat with toxin or benzos.

Hint #1

Associated with long-term neuroleptic use.

Hint #2

Like "Yawning Man" but with eye signs.

Meige Syndrome

Characterized by lingual, facial, and oromandibular spasms, Meige syndrome, named after French neurologist Henri Meige who first described it in 1910, disproportionately affects women and with an onset typically in their 50s. Oromandibular spasms along with blepharospasm are prominent as these patients most commonly experience forced jaw opening or closure, protrusion of the tongue, lip retraction or pursing, and platysma spasm, though can also have bruxism and/or jaw deviation. Much more rarely, these patients can develop torticollis as well as limbs and truncal dystonias that can produce tremor. Though the majority of cases are idiopathic, ~25% have been found to be linked to the use of long-term neuroleptic medications. Ongoing research is looking into potential associations with genetic mutations and other movement disorders.

Meige syndrome can be distinguished clinically from the less common Brueghel syndrome as those with the latter have an isolated gaped mouth from oromandibular spasm. Interestingly this syndrome is named after a painting by a sixteenth century Dutch Renaissance painter Pieter Brueghel the Elder entitled "Yawning Man" or ironically "De Gaper" in Dutch due to the resemblance of these patients to the painting.

Treatment is mostly similar to any other form of focal dystonia. Botulinum toxin injections play a pivotal role. Other options include anticholinergics, tetrabenazine, baclofen, and benzodiazepines.

82

• • • • •

Postinfection/vaccination,
Multifocal inflammation,
Acute onset before 18,
Monophasic lesions seen.

Hint #1

Like MS, but all at once.

Hint #2

Ask Dr. Hurst about the worst kind.

Acute Disseminated Encephalomyelitis

Acute disseminated encephalomyelitis (ADEM) is a monophasic illness characterized by multifocal CNS inflammation and demyelination that occurs primarily in children below 10 years of age (~80%), though it can occur in teenage years and very rarely in adulthood. In the majority of cases of ADEM, a preceding recent immunological stressor can be identified, usually in the form of a routine vaccination (postvaccinal ADEM) or a childhood illness such as influenza or mononucleosis (post-exanthematous ADEM).

The exact pathogenesis of ADEM is unknown, though it is generally thought that the large autoimmune response is due to a cross-reactivity of the initial stressor humoral or cell-mediated response, with myelin autoantigens such as myelin basic protein or myelin oligodendrocyte protein. A more neurologically devastating form of ADEM is acute hemorrhagic leukoencephalitis, also known as Hurst disease or acute necrotizing hemorrhagic encephalomyelitis, occurring several days after the resolution of a preceding illness, with the patient developing high fever, altered mentation, seizure, and coma.

In cases of ADEM, MRI will show multifocal areas of T2/FLAIR hyperintensity, often enhancing on T1 Gad sequences with a partial ring-like appearance (open ring sign) with the open part facing the cortex. The CSF analysis of ADEM can look considerably like multiple sclerosis, showing a lymphocyte-predominant pleocytosis, elevated protein, and positive bands. It is its monophasic nature along with the history of immune stressor that help differentiate ADEM from multiple sclerosis.

All patients with ADEM must be tested for anti-MOG (myelin oligodendrocyte) and AQP4 antibodies (for NMO).

Treatment options include high dose IV steroids. For patients with limited response, IVIG and plasma exchange can be considered as well.

83

· · · · ·

Early onset poor cognition,
Unequal rigid condition,
Apraxia and alien limb,
Post-frontal atrophy within.

Hint #1

Unsure, ask Dr. Strangelove.

Hint #2

Find the answer, get a "plus."

Corticobasal Degeneration

An atypical Parkinsonian syndrome, corticobasal degeneration (CBD) is a neurodegenerative disease characterized by asymmetric focal cortical atrophy in the parasagittal regions, especially in the peri-Rolandic gyri (the areas directly adjacent to the central sulcus). It more commonly affects patients in their 40s to 70s, most commonly in their 60s.

CBD is mainly considered to be a tauopathy. Tau is a normally expressed protein in neurons, which is thought to play a role in stabilizing microtubules. Tau microtubule-binding protein can have three repeats (3R) or four repeats (4R). Normally, 3R and 4R are present in an equal ratio but this ratio is off in neurodegeneration. CBD is predominantly a 4R tauopathy.

The large territory of multitract atrophy produces not only an asymmetric akinetic-rigid movement disorder, but also significant cognitive and sensory impairment. Patients commonly first complain of unilateral hand and arm clumsiness in which rigidity and bradykinesia are found on exam. These patients often also experience cortical sensory loss, myoclonus, resting and action tremor, uncontrollable limb movements, cognitive impairment, aphasia, and apraxia in that limb. On exam these patients are also often found to have increased reflexes, a present Babinski sign, and loss of postural reflexes. As the disease course progresses, signs and symptoms become bilateral, and cognitive impairment becomes more prominent.

Cognitive impairment presents in approximately half of those first presenting with symptoms of CBD, and develops in ~70% of patients over the course of the disease. These patients not only develop significant impairment in executive function and memory, which are common in other neurodegenerative diseases such as Alzheimer's disease, progressive supranuclear palsy, and frontotemporal dementia, but also develop expressive aphasia, helping to differentiate it. Though language comprehension is usually preserved through most of the disease course, as CBD progresses, patients often also develop a receptive aphasia and some progress to complete mutism.

Apraxia also develops in approximately half of patients with CBD. The most common type of apraxia in these patients is ideomotor apraxia, which is the inability to "act out" or perform a skilled gesture when commanded to do so, for example, imitating combing one's hair, lighting a match, or locking a door.

Approximately 30% of patients with CBD develop a phenomenon known as alien limb syndrome characterized by irrepressible involuntary movements in one arm, and a sensation that the affected limb is foreign to them. Interestingly, this phenomenon is also known as Dr. Strangelove syndrome after the famous 1964 Stanley Kubrick film *Dr. Strangelove*, in which the main character's right arm appears to take on a mind of its own, repeatedly trying to choke the main character or give a Nazi salute.

Asymmetric atrophy of the frontoparietal lobe can be seen on CT and MRI, in addition to frontoparietal and basal ganglionic hypometabolism on PET scan and asymmetric frontoparietal hypoperfusion on SPECT.

84

• • • • •

Location, hertz, and amplitude,
Will change with anxiousness or mood,
Distraction will suppress movement,
Some subconscious, and some intent.

Psychogenic Tremor

Psychogenic tremor is a type of nonphysiological tremor. It often occurs in patients with underlying psychiatric conditions such as major depression, anxiety, or PTSD. Psychogenic tremors can take many forms and change location, frequency, and character, which is a helpful distinguishing factor from organic forms of tremor.

Though the signs of psychogenic tremor are vast, it usually presents in one limb (the dominant hand), is irregular in nature, with less stereotyped movement than organic tremors. Psychogenic tremors also often change amplitude and frequency throughout the clinical exam and are "distractible." Distractibility describes the character of a tremor changing when the clinician "distracts" the patient from the tremor by having him/her perform a challenging cognitive task or has the patient concentrate on a task on the contralateral side of the tremor. A distractible tremor will change in character and often subside when attention is concentrated elsewhere. Another common distinguishing characteristic of psychogenic tremor from types of physiological tremor is the changing location of the tremors with focal suppression. This is elicited clinically when a provider restrains the tremoring area, for example, the right hand. Immediately or shortly after restraint of the hand, the "tremor" is then seen to move more proximally to the shoulder or to another body limb altogether, a phenomenon known as *tremor chasing*. Entrainment is also a sign that can be elicited by clever bedside examination. It indicates change in the frequency of the tremor when the patient is asked to perform a repetitive task with the other hand at a certain frequency.

Just like any other functional neurological disorder, it is important to explain the diagnosis to the patient. Treatment will require a multidisciplinary approach with psychiatry and psychology. Psychotherapy like cognitive behavioral therapy (CBT) plays an important role in the management.

85

• • • • •

Change in character without,
Insight, infarcts, fever, about,
Dement, impulse, and over eat,
CSF clean, brain incomplete.

Hint #1

Hopefully getting the right answer is not *out of character*.

Hint #2

Most common type in this "younger" population.

267

Frontotemporal Dementia

Though less common than vascular dementia, Alzheimer's disease, and dementia with Lewy bodies, frontotemporal dementia (FTD) is the most common cause of dementia in those younger than 60 years old, with most cases occurring from 45 to 65 years of age. There are two major types of FTD, behavioral FTD and primary progressive aphasia; and three subtypes of primary progressive aphasia (nonfluent agrammatic, semantic, and logopenic), grouped by their predominant features. Behavioral FTD (bvFTD) has prominent personality and behavioral changes, as well as executive function impairment. Primary progressive aphasia (PPA) is characterized by a predominant language impairment.

From a pathological standpoint, the disease associated with the clinical spectrum of FTD is called FTLD (frontotemporal lobar degeneration). The majority of FTLD cases are characterized by either (1) abnormal tau protein formation and deposition (tauopathy), or (2) abnormal deposition of TAR DNA-binding protein 43 (TDP-43 proteinopathy). Additionally, CHMP2B-related ubiquitinated inclusions or the presence of the "fused in sarcoma" (FUS) gene may be present. Cases of bvFTD are caused by either TDP-43 proteinopathy or tauopathy. Whereas most cases of nonfluent agrammatic PPA (nfaPPA) are caused by tauopathy, semantic variant PPA (svPPA) is caused by TDP-43 proteinopathy, and logopenic variant PPA (lvPPA) has underlying Alzheimer's disease. There is also a known familial component to FTD with ~25–50% of cases having FTD also present in at least one first-degree relative. The most common genetic mutations associated with familial FTD are C9orf72 (also commonly found in familial amyotrophic lateral sclerosis), MAPT, and GPRN.

The signs of bvFTD are predominantly changes in the patient's character and behavior, with no or very mild impairment in memory or spatial skills. These patients often present with impulsivity, disinhibition, decreased social awareness, aberrant social conduct, inappropriate joking or laughter, oral fixation, declining personal hygiene, or changes in sexual and diet interests. They also typically lack both insight and concern about their personality changes. In conversation, these patients often show perseveration, fixed or inflexible ideation, blunted emotions, and stereotyped mannerisms and behaviors. Though language impairment is uncommonly present in the early stages of bvFTD, signs including echolalia, verbal stereotyping, and decreased speech quantity can occur with disease progression. Additional motor, sensory, and reflex changes are typically absent, though these patients do often develop recurrence of primitive reflexes (also known as frontal release signs), most commonly palmomental, grasp, and snout. For the majority of patients with FTD, visuospatial coordination remains unimpaired. In bvFTD, atrophy of the frontal and temporal lobes can be seen on CT and MRI.

Those with nfaPPA typically present with difficulty producing speech, inappropriate word use, or word order, and progressively worsening grammar. These patients often develop progressive anomia, speech simplification, apraxia of speech, and eventually become mute. Interestingly, however, those with nfaPPA have relatively preserved language comprehension and retain the ability to follow simple commands, though complex commands may become difficult. Additionally, late in nfaFTD, patients also often develop behavior changes, characteristic of bvFTD. Neuroimaging of those with nfaFTD will most commonly show left perisylvian atrophy (mainly fronto-insular).

The primary signs of svPPA are most typically anomia, impaired picture naming and single-word comprehension, difficulty remembering distant life events, in the presence of fluent, normal cadenced speech, and unimpaired short-term memory. This is also evidenced clinically by the presence of compensatory semantic paraphrasias and significant difficulty with categorical fluency testing, such as asking the patient to list items in a category such as animals, foods, or furniture. Like in all forms of PPA, behavior changes may develop; however they are not predominate. On both CT and MRI, these patients most often have atrophy of the left anterior temporal lobe with or without atrophy of the right anterior temporal lobe.

In lvPPA, patients have speech that is particularly lacking descriptive detail, has frequent word-finding pauses, and use common phonemic paraphrasias, using or substituting a similar sounding but incorrect word for an intended word ("cook" substituted for "book," or "computer" pronounced" conpuner"). These patients often have difficulty with sentence repetition. In these patients, neuroimaging will typically show left parietal and posterior temporal atrophy.

Motor neuron disease (MND) can precede or follow the development of FTD, especially the bvFTD. The most common genetic cause of FTD-MND spectrum is C9orf72 mutation. The characteristics of MND in FTD-MND are similar to that of classic ALS with some differences. Bulbar symptoms and pseudobulbar affect are more common in FTD-MND compared to classic ALS.

86

· · · · ·

Often found in younger more,
From lining cells of fourth of four,
Depressed mentation, third dilate,
Resection or irradiate.

Hint #1

Can spread through CSF.

Hint #2

Think perivascular pseudorosettes.

Ependymoma

Ependymomas are glial tumors that arise from the ependymal cells that line the ventricles and the central canal of the spinal cord, mostly located in the fourth ventricle. These tumors commonly affect children aged 1–5 years, though can be found in young adults. Like astrocytomas, ependymomas are graded based on histological characteristics, with grade 1 representing subapendy-moma/myxopapillary ependymoma, grade 2 representing ependy-moma, and grade 3 representing anaplastic ependymoma.

Those with an ependymoma usually present with signs and symptoms of obstructive hydrocephalus, namely, impaired con-sciousness, headache, nausea, and imbalance, as well as cranial nerve palsy.

Given that ependymomas can spread through CSF, contrasted imaging of the complete neuroaxis is important. In addition to contrast-enhancement of the solid portions of the tumor, hemor-rhages, calcifications, and cysts can also be present, though biopsy is needed for definitive diagnosis.

The initial treatment of choice is safe maximal surgical resec-tion. For cases with gross total resection, adjuvant radiation can be used as well. For patients with subtotal resection, both radiation and chemotherapy can be used. In patients where there is imaging and/or clinical evidence of dissemination along the neuroaxis, focused radiation of the neuroaxis is required.

Overall, the prognosis is poor with ~50–70% 10-year survival.

87

• • • • •

Disorder more in young boys which,
Are seen to have grunting and twitch,
Most will tic, few say obscene,
So up alpha-2 or blunt dopamine.

Hint #1

These patients often develop mental illness in adulthood.

Hint #2

Eye blinking is the most common initial symptom.

Tourette Syndrome

Named after George Gilles de la Tourette who published an in-depth description of the disorder in 1885, Tourette syndrome (TS) is a pediatric tic disorder with a 3:1 male predominance. Though there is ample evidence that tic disorders are often familial, research has not found a definitive gene associated with the inheritance of TS. Many theories exist about the pathogenesis of TS, most of which center around the hypothesis that there is some sort of dopamine abnormality in the striatum, a pathogenesis that is supported by the fact that tics more commonly occur in patients with dopamine irregularity such as patients with Parkinson disease or Huntington disease.

Tics can be both motor and vocal/phonic. Motor tics are brief, purposeless, rapid movements that occur with otherwise normal motor activity. Tics can be broadly divided into *simple* and *complex* tics. Simply motor tics can involve any area of the body and characterized by any short-lived movement such as a blink or neck movement, or a sustained contraction, such as tensing of the forearm or abdomen. Simple vocal tics are similar to simple motor tics in brevity and diversity, often represented as a sniff, cough, click, grunt, or throat-clearing. Complex motor tics involve more complicated motor movements such as pantomiming, tapping, or touching; while complex vocal tics can take the form of the statement of purposeless words or phrases. Both motor and vocal tics are often stereotyped actions that are repetitive, and patients often express an urge to perform the tic that is relieved after performing it.

Patients with TS develop both motor and vocal tics, experienced multiple times a day, prior to the age of 21 and lasting for more than one year. Those with TS experience considerable impairment and distress due to their tics. There is considerable psychological comorbidity in TS with ~50% of patients showing clinical signs of obsessive-compulsive disorder (more common in females with TS) and/or attention deficit hyperactivity disorder (more common in males with TS).

Mild tics do not require pharmacologic treatment. For severe tics that cause significant physical and functional impairment, the first-line treatment is comprehensive behavioral intervention for tics (CBIT). Pharmacologic options include guanfacine, tetrabenazine, and deutetrabenazine. For tics involving violent neck movements, botulinum toxin injections are indicated.

88

• • • • •

Hand contraction, distal weak,
Bulbar involvement, hairdo meek,
Autosomal dominant,
Cardiac symptoms prominent.

Hint #1

Most also have cardiac abnormalities.

Hint #2

Tap on their hand, see a sustained contraction.

Myotonic Dystrophy

The most common form of muscular dystrophy in adults, myotonic dystrophy (MD) is an autosomal dominant neuromuscular disease caused by the trinucleotide expansion of CTG repeats. The location of these CTG repeats differs between types of MD with the chromosome 19 gene DMPK (dystrophia-myotonica protein kinase) being the culprit gene in myotonic dystrophy type 1 (DM-1 aka Steinert's disease), and the chromosome 3 gene ZnFP9 (zinc finger protein 9) being the culprit gene in myotonic dystrophy type 2 (DM-2). A greater number of CTG repeats predicts an earlier onset of disease.

Signs of DM-1 can occur at any age, including the neonatal period, and generally consist of progressive distal greater than proximal muscle weakness, along with facial, nuchal, and bulbar weakness. Patients with DM-1 characteristically develop footdrop and hand weakness. These patients often end up having some extent of frontal balding. The myotonia that develops can often easily be elicited with tongue or thenar percussion, or asking the patient to quickly release after a sustained firm hand grip. Additionally, however, those with adult-onset DM-1 have a significant risk of mortality by respiratory (~40%) and cardiac failure (~30%), and ~25% have atrial flutter or fibrillation, and 2–30% die of sudden cardiac death. Those with DM-1 have higher rates of insulin resistance and cataracts than the average population.

The subtypes of DM-1 are divided by age and severity (congenital-onset DM-1, childhood or juvenile onset DM-1, adult-onset DM-1, and mild DM-1). Adult-onset DM-1 is the most common type and is characterized by the signs/symptoms listed above. Congenital-onset DM-1 is characterized by profound muscle weakness, hypotonia, and near-global developmental delay. Childhood/juvenile-onset DM-1 is less severe but characterized by muscle weakness, cognitive and behavioral impairment, and ~10% develop cardiomyopathy or heart failure. Also known as proximal myotonic myopathy (PROMM) DM-2 is a rarer and less severe form that affects proximal muscles greater than distal muscles, and is usually found in adults, rarely children, and never in neonates.

Needle EMG demonstrates the presence of myotonic discharges that fire at 20–150 Hz with waxing and waning amplitude. These discharges sound like a motorcycle engine. The presence of myotonic discharges is not specific to MD though. Genetic testing must be performed to confirm the diagnosis.

Most of the care is supportive. For patients with significant myotonic symptoms, mexiletine can be used for symptomatic relief.

89

• • • • •

Double vision, eye outward,
Due to a clot that has occurred,
Ataxia and tremor see,
On opposite side of body.

Hint #1

Do not get distracted *mid*-thought.

Hint #2

Friends with Weber and Claude.

Benedikt Syndrome (Medial/Ventral Midbrain Infarction)

Also called *paramedian midbrain syndrome,* Benedikt syndrome is a lacunar stroke syndrome of the base and tegmentum of the midbrain, named after Austrian neurologist Moiz Benedikt, who detailed the signs in a lecture in 1889.

Benedikt syndrome is caused by occlusion of either the posterior cerebral artery or the paramedian penetrating branches of the basilar artery. The territory of infarct usually involves the red nucleus (including the fibers from the superior cerebellar peduncle), fascicles of the oculomotor nerve, the substantia nigra, and the corticospinal tract.

Signs of Benedikt syndrome often include ipsilateral oculomotor nerve palsy (CN3) causing the affected eye to be down and out at rest with the weakness of adduction and elevation. Contralateral hemiataxia and tremor occur from the involvement of the red nucleus and superior cerebellar peduncle fibers.

Additionally, contralateral hemichorea and athetosis can also occur because of involvement of the substantia nigra, and patients can have contralateral hemiparesis from the involvement of the corticospinal tract.

90

• • • • •

Middle age tumor calcified,
And up-close see egg served fried,
Deletes on chrome' 1 and 19,
And mutations in IDH seen.

Hint #1

Look for chicken-wire vasculature.

Hint #2

A relatively rare type of glioma.

Oligodendroglioma

Most commonly occurring in middle age (35–45 years old), oligo-dendrogliomas are the third most common type of glial cell tumor, representing only 1–5% of all primary brain tumors. These patients commonly present with seizures; however, they can have a wide variety of signs and symptoms depending on tumor location, size, and grade.

On MRI, oligodendrogliomas are most commonly found to be supratentorial, in the cortical and subcortical tissue with a frontal lobe predominance. They are very rarely found in the cerebellum, brainstem, or spinal cord. Intratumoral calcification and cysts are common, though central necrosis is not. Histologically, oligoden-drogliomas have round nuclei with perinuclear clearing (fried egg appearance) with small delicate blood vessels (chicken wire vasculature).

In the WHO classification of diffuse gliomas, oligodendroglio-mas are identified by a combination of co-deletions in chromo-some 1p and 19q and a mutation in the enzyme isocitrate dehydrogenase 1 or 2 (IDH1 or IDH2).

The mainstay of treatment is maximal surgical resection. For Gr III oligodendrogliomas, surgical resection must be followed by radiation and adjuvant chemotherapy. Chemotherapy options include temozolomide or PCV (procarbazine, lomustine, and vin-cristine). The median survival of patients with chemotherapy is up to 20 years.

91

• • • • •

First atax/spasticity,
Then dementia late will be,
A prion family history,
Mutation in PRNP.

Hint #1

High RT-QuIC false-negative rate.

Hint #1

Death in 5–10 years.

Gerstmann–Straussler–Scheinker Syndrome

Gerstmann-Straussler-Scheinker syndrome (GSS) is a very rare type of prion disease most commonly inherited via an autosomal dominant pattern with mutations in the PRNP gene at codons 102 (most common), 105, 117, and 198, located on chromosome 20. Though the clinical manifestations of GSS depend on the mutation inherited, most of these patients will develop symptoms of ataxia, spasticity, and rigidity in the early phases of the disease, as well as dementia in the later stages. Those with GSS typically develop symptoms in their 40s to 70s, which progress rapidly, with death typically 5-10 years after onset.

Due to the high heterogeneity of GSS, diagnostic CSF testing is relatively insensitive with RT-QuIC assay studies showing high numbers of false negative results. Additionally, with EEG and neuroimaging showing nonspecific findings, diagnosis is reliant on clinical history and physical exam. In addition to the typical histological findings of CJD, neuropathologically, these patients will have a cerebellar predominant amyloid plaque deposition, though definitive diagnosis is made through genetic testing for the PRNP gene.

92

• • • • •

At first with trouble sleeping then,
Atax and then dement begin,
Sleep study shows loss of REM,
PRNP prognosis grim.

Hint #1

Look for thalamic atrophy.

Hint #2

Most have significant dysautonomia.

Fatal Familial Insomnia

Like Gerstmann–Straussler–Scheinker syndrome (GSS) and subtypes of Creutzfeldt–Jakob disease (CJD), fatal familial insomnia (FFI) is a very rare familial prion disease passed by autosomal dominant inheritance, though sporadic cases have been found (sFI). Also, like GSS and CJD, FFI is caused by a mutation in the PRNP gene on chromosome 20, specifically co-mutation at codons 178 and 129.

Signs and symptoms of both FFI and sFI typically occur between ages 40 and 70 and present as a progressive sleep impairment with insomnia, a dream-like wake state, and dream enactment (oneiric stupor). The dream enactment of oneiric stupor is different from that of REM behavioral disorder (RBD) because these patients usually stay in a transition stage between wakefulness and stage I sleep. They have poor sleep wave architecture with the absence of deeper stages of sleep. In addition to sleep dysfunction, those with fatal insomnia also have significant dysautonomia characterized by temperature, heart rate, blood pressure dysregulation, hyperhidrosis, and hyperlacrimation. This constellation of symptoms is referred to as Agrypnia excitata. The other major differentials for Agrypnia excitata include alcohol withdrawal and Morvan syndrome.

Like GSS, cases of FFI and sFI can be difficult to reliably detect by CSF as RT-QuIC testing has low sensitivities and high false negative rates.

Neuropathological examination of these patients will show focal atrophy and gliosis of the thalamus with scattered focal cerebral spongiosis. Sequencing of the PRNP gene provides a definitive diagnosis. FFI is a lethal progressive neurodegenerative disorder with a mean duration of 13 months.

93

• • • • •

Symptoms of stroke, seizure, dement,
High lactate, fibers present,
In the young symptoms display,
Mutated mtDNA.

Hint #1

Strokes are most common at <40 years old.

Hint #2

These fibers are ragged and colorful.

Mitochondrial Encephalopathy, Lactic Acidosis, and Stroke-Like Episodes Syndrome (MELAS)

Mitochondrial encephalopathy, lactic acidosis, and stroke-like episodes syndrome (MELAS) is a maternally inherited disorder caused primarily by a mutation in the tRNA of the MT-TL1 gene of mitochondrial DNA, accounting for ~80% of cases. Many other causal mutations have been found, most of which are mutations in tRNA genes, and all impairing mitochondrial protein synthesis. The pathogenesis of the stroke-like symptoms is not well understood; however, it has been proposed that those with MELAS may have impaired blood flow due to the overabundance of mitochondria in the small arterioles and capillaries of their neuro-vasculature, or impaired vascular metabolism.

The three clinical features after which MELAS is named are required for diagnosis. The stroke-like symptoms typically occur prior to age 40, and though the signs appear clinically identical to those of acute cerebral ischemia, the cortical lesions seen on MRI do not conform to typical cerebrovascular territories. The encephalopathy associated with MELAS often appears clinically as dementia and/or seizures. The mitochondrial dysfunction of MELAS results in lactic acidosis and/or ragged-red fibers on muscle biopsy. In addition to these three core clinical features of MELAS, two or more of the following must be present: vomiting, recurrent headaches, and normal early childhood development. Though not required for diagnosis, those with MELAS also often experience myoclonus, myopathic weakness, ataxia, hearing loss, and stunted growth. Definitive diagnosis can be confirmed by identifying one of the many known causal mtDNA mutations in the blood.

Stroke-like episodes in MELAS are often triggered by seizures; hence aggressive treatment of seizures with IV anti-seizure medications like levetiracetam, phenytoin, or lacosamide is required. Arginine supplementation has also been used although no conclusive evidence is available.

94

• • • • •

Myoclonus and seizures,
Ataxic movements key features,
Passed from mother fibers red,
mtDNA change'd.

Hint #1

Most have an A-to-G mutation.

Hint #2

The name is an acronym describing the three main clinical findings.

MERRF Syndrome

Myoclonic epilepsy with ragged-red fibers (MERRF) syndrome, also called Fukahara syndrome, is a very rare maternally inherited mitochondrial disorder caused by a mutation in mitochondrial DNA. Approximately 80% of cases of MERRF are caused by an A-to-G mutation in the mitochondrial MT-TK gene, encoding tRNA.

Clinical features of MERRF, as the name suggests, are myoclonus, generalized seizures, and a muscle biopsy showing ragged-red fibers, after normal early childhood development. Other common signs and symptoms of MERRF include ataxia, muscle weakness, hearing loss, optic atrophy, cognitive impairment often to the point of dementia, short stature, peripheral neuropathy, cardiac conduction irregularities, and lactic acidosis that causes abdominal pain and vomiting.

95

• • • • •

Post a blast or head impact,
lights too bright, slow to react,
some throw up, stumble about,
imaging clean, sit this one out.

Hint #1

Wear your helmet.

Hint #2

Usually resolved in <1 month.

Concussion

The definition of concussion has changed many times over the last 50 years; however, in general, concussion is a subset of mild traumatic brain injury and represents a traumatically induced transient disturbance in neuronal function that cannot be otherwise explained. Though the exact pathophysiology of concussion is unknown, it is thought that during a concussion a force is delivered to the brain by any of multiple modalities (e.g., physical force such as head impact or pressure force such as blast injury) that creates a stretch of the neurons, which in turn disrupts neuronal functions and communication. This disruption also results in some extent of direct structural cell injury and impairs their ability to repair themselves, making them more vulnerable to a second and more harmful later concussion. Though most concussions occur due to a physical force impacting the head and translation of that force to the brain, blast concussions are common in those that serve in the military, and it is generally thought to occur when a nearby explosion changes the intra and extracranial pressures and causes an acceleration force to the head and brain, resulting in neuronal damage.

Concussion is a clinical diagnosis. To date there are no widely used or definitively sensitive or specific tests available. Common symptoms of concussion are headache, dizziness, fatigue, "fogginess," and mood changes. In athletics, providers use the preparticipation physical examination (PPE) to serve as a baseline evaluation that logs a balance and cognitive evaluation, prior history of head injury, premorbid conditions such as mood or learning disorders, and headache disorders. The tested components of the PPE overlap significantly with the assessments that can be performed and compared later, either on the field or in a care provider's office, when a concussion is suspected.

It is generally accepted for an athlete to be removed from play if a potentially concussive event resulted in any loss of consciousness, imbalance, or coordination issues, as well as a blank stare on the player's face, and it is recommended to keep the player out of the game until evaluated in an environment that is as distraction-free as possible.

The symptoms that the patient/athlete reports along with the reevaluation comparison to the PPE is the most sensitive indicator of concussion. Standard evaluation tools, such as the commonly used sports concussion assessment tool (SCAT5), incorporate exam findings, cognitive and balance testing, and a symptom checklist to help assess the likelihood of concussion. Athletes found unlikely to have experienced a concussion are often allowed to continue sports participation, while athletes found to have probable or definite concussion are immediately removed from play and no same-day play is recommended.

The vestibular/ocular motor screening (VOMS) tool can be particularly helpful in diagnosing concussion as approximately 67%–77% of patients with sports-related concussion will have symptoms of vestibular (balance) impairment, and approximately 45% will have impairment in eye movement and function.

Approximately 80%–90% of concussed adolescent and young adult patients experience a complete resolution of their new post-concussive symptoms within two weeks after the event without treatment, though younger adolescent athletes may take slightly longer (two to four weeks).

96

• • • • •

Illness in kids, when hot half brain,
With seizures that post-med remain,
Result in weakness on one side,
Final treat, half brain debride.

Hint #1

Most experience epilepsia partialis continua.

Hint #2

Highly resistant to medication. Hemispherectomy?

Rasmussen Syndrome/Encephalitis

First described by Canadian neurologist and neurosurgeon Theodore Rasmussen and colleagues in 1958, Rasmussen syndrome (RS), also called Rasmussen encephalitis, is a rare, severe form of chronic childhood neuroinflammatory disease producing drug-resistant focal epilepsy, most often resulting in progressive hemiparesis. Most cases of RS occur in children between ages 3 and 15, though RS has also been seen in adults (~10%). The etiology of RS is unknown and thought to be sporadic.

Though the seizures seen in RS can be both focal and generalized, ~50%–90% of these patients experience epilepsia partialis continua. The seizures seen in RS are highly resistant to medication. As seizures become more frequent, neurological deterioration begins, most often in the form of progressive hemiparesis, cognitive impairment, hemianopia, and aphasia if seizures involve the dominant hemisphere. After the first onset of seizures, most patients with RS progress to the point of severe permanent physical and cognitive disability within 12–16 months. Histopathologically, those with RS are found to have significant unilateral neuronal destruction and T-lymphocytic infiltrative gliosis of the cortex, as well as tissue necrosis and atrophy, meningeal inflammation, and perivascular cuffing. Though very rarely, cases of bilateral RS have been documented.

Cerebrospinal fluid analysis in patients with RS is highly variable, with no sensitive or specific antibodies currently known, and should be used to rule out CNS infection. On MRI, ipsilateral caudate atrophy is often the first appreciable sign of RS, prior to unilateral generalized hemispheric atrophy seen on T1, and unilateral hyperintensity seen on T2. Diffusion restriction can also be seen unilaterally, though usually no contrast-enhancement is present.

The most effective treatment for the refractory epilepsy in RS is hemispherectomy.

97

· · · · ·

First the trunk, and then in limb,
Atax with altered ATM,
In kids with vessel dilation,
Poor immune and cancer in.

Hint #1

Most also develop immunodeficiency and malignancy.

Hint #2

Autosomal recessively inherited.

Ataxia-Telangiectasia

Ataxia-telangiectasia (AT), also called Louis-Bar syndrome, is the most common inherited childhood progressive ataxia in most countries, most often seen during infancy, in ages 1–3. Inherited in an autosomal recessive pattern, AT is caused by mutation of the ATM gene, located on chromosome 11q22–23.

The signs of AT typically begin with truncal ataxia, seen in toddlerhood with difficulty sitting up or excessively unstable gait. Ataxia later becomes evident in the limbs, while the development of oculomotor apraxia and dysarthria often hinders early school years performance. Telangiectasias often develop a few years after the onset of ataxia, and most often affect the conjunctivae and sun-exposed areas such as the ears and face.

Most patients with AT will also have some degree of immuno-deficiency, most commonly seen as a low IgA or IgG and a low CD4 cell count. Because of this, many patients with AT experience recurrent pulmonary and sinus infections, resulting in long-term pulmonary morbidities such as interstitial lung disease or bronchiectasis. Approximately one-third of those with AT will develop a malignancy during their lifetime, most common of which are lymphoma and leukemia, which usually develop prior to age 20. Though less common, patients with AT are also much more likely than the general population to develop solid tumors such as breast, ovarian, gastric, liver, and skin cancers, these usually developing later in life.

Bloodwork testing for immunodeficiency can be helpful in diagnosis, specifically looking for low IgA, IgG, and IgE. Levels of IgM can be variable. Additionally, ~90% of those with AT will have elevated alpha-fetoprotein, though this is nonspecific. MRI findings are usually absent until many years after onset of signs and symptoms; however when present, cerebellar atrophy, especially the cerebellar vermis, is prominent. Because of the large number of ATM gene mutations that can cause AT, genetic testing is not routinely used, but Western immunoblot analysis should show very low or absent levels of ATM protein.

98

• • • • •

Seizures in kids age 3–6,
Affects mostly autonomics,
Most throw up, urine cannot keep,
Occipital spikes occur in sleep.

Hint #1

MRI is normal.

Hint #2

Named after a Greek epileptologist.

Panayiotopoulos Syndrome

Panayiotopoulos syndrome (PS) was first described by and later named after Greek epileptologist Chrysostomos Panayiotopoulos in the late 1980s. A common benign childhood epilepsy, PS is estimated to make up 13% of all cases of epilepsy in children aged 3–6 years, though it can be seen also during teenage years. It is also known as early-onset childhood occipital epilepsy as opposed to the late-onset childhood occipital epilepsy known as Gastaut syndrome. They are all subtypes of benign focal epilepsies of childhood.

Those with PS experience seizures that begin with autonomic signs (~80%), most commonly vomiting (~70%), but may include pallor, flushing, mydriasis, or incontinence. These seizures occur during sleep in ~70% of those with PS, and if awake, most will report feeling sick and then vomiting, while ~20% of patients will experience a syncope-like event (ictal syncope) and lose consciousness during the seizure. In some cases, this may be the only clinical sign present. In ~40% of cases, these autonomic seizures will last >30 minutes, constituting autonomic status epilepticus. After the onset of autonomic symptoms, ~60% of patients will experience head version and unilateral gaze, while ~40% will experience a hemi-clonic or generalized clonic seizure.

The characteristic interictal EEG finding is the presence of occipital spikes with the peculiar morphology similar to the centrotemporal spikes of Rolandic epilepsy. These spikes have an initial small positive spike, followed by a large negative spike, then a positive slow wave larger than the positive spike and then a negative slow wave, smaller than the negative spike. These spikes often become more obvious with eyes closed, called fixation-off sensitivity (FOS). MRI in these patients is typically normal. Complete remission often occurs one to two years after onset, and most patients experience five or less total seizures. Most patients do not require anti-seizure medications, except for those with very frequent seizures.

99

● ● ● ● ●

Often found at fork'd path,
And 5% of healthy hath,
Found by mistake, before goes pop,
Some cranial nerve push atop.

Hint #1

Most commonly found in the circle of Willis.

Hint #2

Can cause CN 3 palsy or bitemporal hemianopsia.

Unruptured Intracranial Aneurysm

Unruptured intracranial aneurysms are found in ~3–5% of healthy adults, with ~85–90% never becoming symptomatic or rupture. The overall five-year risk of aneurysmal rupture is ~3% and is highly influenced by vascular risk factors such as smoking, hypertension, and psychostimulant use, as well as nonmodifiable risk factors such as aneurysm size, prior aneurysmal subarachnoid hemorrhage, and female sex. Additionally, those with certain genetic and connective tissue disorders such as Ehlers–Danlos syndrome, Marfan syndrome, and polycystic kidney disease are predisposed to the formation of intracranial aneurysms. It is estimated that ~20% of patients with a history of a ruptured aneurysm also have an unruptured aneurysm at a separate location.

Intracranial aneurysms are most commonly found at areas of artery bifurcation. The most common location for intracranial aneurysms (ruptured and unruptured) is within the circle of Willis, with ~35% located in the anterior communicating artery, ~30% at the junction of the posterior communicating artery and internal carotid artery, and ~20% arising from the middle cerebral artery. Unruptured intracranial aneurysms can cause headache and cranial nerve compression. The most commonly affected cranial nerve is the oculomotor nerve (CN3) being compressed by a posterior communicating artery aneurysm causing an ipsilateral oculomotor nerve palsy. A bitemporal hemianopsia can also be caused by compression of the optic chiasm by an aneurysm of the anterior communication artery.

Two large prospective studies – ISUIA (international study of unruptured intracranial aneurysms) and UCAS (unruptured cerebral aneurysms study) provided data on the natural history of unruptured aneurysms. Aneurysms below 7 mm in size are considered to be at low risk for rupture. The five-year risk of rupture increases with the increasing size of the aneurysm. Aneurysms larger than 25 mm have a 40% risk of rupture. In addition, the location of the aneurysm also predicts the risk of rupture with those located in the posterior circulation being at the highest risk of rupture.

As far as management is concerned, those decisions must be individualized based on a patient's five-year risk of rupture and perioperative morbidity and mortality. There are no randomized clinical trials that have studied this. Based on a cost-effectiveness study, the treatment of aneurysms <10 mm in size with no prior history of SAH led to worse outcomes, whereas the treatment of larger aneurysms with prior history of SAH improved outcomes.

100

• • • • •

Strokes in young, through families passed,
First migraines, slow thinking last,
With white disease and lacunes seen,
and mutation of the Notch 3 gene.

Hint #1

Look for hyperintensity in the anterior temporal lobes.

Hint #2

Known by a long acronym.

Cerebral Autosomal Dominant (or Recessive) Arteriopathy with Subcortical Infarcts and Leukoencephalopathy (CADASIL/CARASIL)

Cerebral autosomal dominant arteriopathy with subcortical infarcts and leukoencephalopathy CADASIL and its recessively inherited version CARASIL are cerebral small-vessel diseases caused by missense mutation in the NOTCH 3 gene located on chromosome 19. Interestingly, this locus is the same as seen in familial hemiplegic migraine, and migraine is the first symptom these patients experience in ~40% of cases in Caucasians. However, migraine prevalence varies widely based on ethnic background, occurring less commonly in those of Asian heritage.

The three main clinical features of CADASIL/CARASIL are migraine with aura, recurrent subcortical ischemic events (stroke and TIA), and progressive cognitive impairment. Migraine is reported in ~50–75% of those with CADASIL/CARASIL, beginning around age 30, the vast majority of which have aura. The subcortical ischemic events most commonly present as a lacunar infarct in patients 20–60 years old (average ~40), and because of the small-vessel predominance, infarcts involving larger vessel territories are rarely and uncertainly attributed to CADASIL/CARASIL. The encephalopathy, as well as the first clinical symptoms, seen in CADASIL/CARASIL can be acute in ~10% of cases, with most episodes of encephalopathy occurring after a migraine attack and consisting of acute confusion and alterations in consciousness, often resolving spontaneously. The cognitive impairment seen in CADASIL/CARASIL disproportionally affects executive function and cognitive processing speed. Both short- and long-term memory is usually preserved, though patients commonly also experience apathy and depression.

In cases of CADASIL/CARASIL, neuroimaging findings on T2 and FLAIR MRI show extensive symmetrical white matter hyperintensity and multiple lacunar infarcts of varying ages. In early stages, white matter hyperintensity in the anterior temporal lobe (~85%) and external capsule (~90%) is particularly sensitive and specific to the diagnosis of CADASIL/CARASIL. Cortical and/or subcortical microhemorrhages are also present in ~50% of cases, and in the late stages of the disease diffuse cerebral atrophy becomes evident.

101

• • • • •

In patients taking long-term meds,
To decrease dopamine,
Irregular, repetitive,
Blink, grimace, movement seen.

Hint #1

Keep those differentials constantly moving.

Hint #2

More commonly seen in the first generation.

Tardive Dyskinesia

Tardive dyskinesia (TD) is a movement disorder characterized by intermittent or continuous hyperkinetic involuntary movements caused by the use of neuroleptic medications, specifically dopamine receptor antagonists, a common mechanism of antipsychotic medications. Though most commonly seen in patients taking dopamine receptor blocking medications, TD can also be seen in patients taking antihistamine and serotonergic medications. These abnormal movements are often most prominent in the orofacial and lingual muscles (lip-smacking, tongue protrusion), though can be seen in the upper- and lower-extremities, nuchal, and truncal muscles. The specific involuntary movements experienced in TD can vary widely between patients, and can include choreiform, dystonic, and stereotyped movements, as well as motor and/or vocal tics and akathisia, particularly in the legs.

In general, the longer a patient is on neuroleptic medications the higher the risk of developing TD. First generation neuroleptic medications are more likely to cause TD than the newer, second-generation antipsychotics. Most patients who stop their causal dopamine receptor-blocking medication experience some degree of recovery, though in most patients the abnormal movements persist despite stopping the offending medication.

The mechanism of TD is not completely understood; however, it is generally thought that the consistent use of dopamine receptor antagonist medications creates an imbalance of dopamine receptor blockade and stimulation in the striatum, resulting in the creation of and inability to stop the abnormal movements. Specifically, the "dopamine hypothesis" proposes that the persistent dopamine receptor blockade results in an upregulation in dopamine receptors and an exaggerated response of these receptors to dopamine.

The first-line treatment of TD is to stop the responsible medication, if possible. Alternatives include lowering the dosage or switching to lower potency medication, for example, switching first-generation antipsychotic to a second-generation antipsychotic. Quetiapine and clozapine have the lowest risk of TD.

If the offending medication cannot be discontinued, treatment options include VMAT2 inhibitors (valbenazine, deutetrabenazine, and tetrabenazine), benzodiazepines, or botulinum toxin injections for focal dystonia.

102

• • • • •

Post-hypoxic no awake,
Cognition is maintained,
But action myoclonus,
Often chronically remained.

Hint #1

You may have a startle response to the correct answer.

Hint #2

Specifically named after its first describers.

Lance–Adams Syndrome

First described by neurologists James Lance and Raymond Adams in 1963, Lance–Adams syndrome (LAS) is a chronic hyperkinetic involuntary movement disorder caused by anoxic brain injury, often secondary to cardiopulmonary arrest. Unlike acute post-anoxic myoclonus, which manifests acutely hours to days after cardiopulmonary arrest, LAS is a chronic sequela appearing days to weeks after the arrest, once the patient has regained consciousness, and often much of their baseline cognitive function. Though cardiac arrest is the most common inciting event, other causes of hypoxic brain injury have been reported to result in LAS such as surgical accidents, attempted suicides, drug overdoses, and asthma attacks.

This chief motor symptom of LAS is myoclonus. In the original article, it was described as intention or action myoclonus, suggesting that it is mainly activated during action. It can also be reflexive and can be elicited by external stimuli such as a startle response (startle myoclonus) or in response to tactile stimuli.

The diagnosis of LAS is made clinically. EEG is often performed as a diagnostic test. EEG may or may not show spikes time-locked to the myoclonus. Polygraphic analysis using EEG and surface-EMG demonstrates that the myoclonus in LAS can be both positive and negative. Jerk-locked back averaging and silent period-locked back averaging can both reveal a small EEG potential preceding the myoclonus when the raw EEG does not show a spike. Overall, the myoclonus can be cortical (spontaneous or reflex) or reticular (spontaneous or reflex) in origin.

Treatment of LAS is difficult and usually disabling myoclonus affecting trunk muscles, causing recurrent falls, persists. Anti-seizure medications that have demonstrated reasonable efficacy against myoclonus include levetiracetam, valproic acid, benzodiazepines, and perampanel.

103

• • • • •

Nothing at rest or with movement,
but after one stands still,
High frequency, low amplitude,
On walking becomes nil.

Hint #1

Only found in the legs.

Hint #2

Symptoms go away when seated.

Orthostatic Tremor

Orthostatic tremor is a relatively rare and unique tremor that is isolated to the legs. This is characterized by a low amplitude, high frequency (14–16 Hz) tremor that is not present while sitting or when reclined but manifests only while the patient is standing still. The amplitude of the movements in orthostatic tremor is often so small that they are invisible to observers, and only appreciable when palpated. These patients often have difficulty initiating their first few steps, but once they start walking, their tremor resolves. These patients often adopt a wide-based cautious gait, with difficulty with tandem gait. Because of the difficult visualization of the tremor due to its low amplitude nature, historically, the symptoms reported by those with orthostatic tremor have been misdiagnosed as hysteria.

Electromyography can be helpful in diagnosis, though is not required, and often shows rhythmic co-contraction of the anterior tibialis and gastrocnemius muscles.

There are no well-established treatment guidelines for management of orthostatic tremor. The most effective medication so far has been clonazepam and other benzodiazepines. Valproate, primidone, and gabapentin have also shown some efficacy. In some refractory cases, deep brain stimulation of ventral intermediate nucleus of thalamus has also been used.

104

• • • • •

In kids who myoclonic-drop,
General spike and wave,
Need ketogenic/valproate,
And helmet for the save.

Hint #1

Must have atonic seizures.

Hint #2

Often outgrown with age.

Doose Syndrome (Myoclonic Astatic Epilepsy)

Doose syndrome, also known as myoclonic astatic epilepsy, is a relatively uncommon childhood epilepsy syndrome first described in 1970 by German physician Dr. Hermann Doose. Accounting for approximately 1% of childhood-onset epilepsies, Doose syndrome often first presents in early to mid-childhood (ages 2–6 years), with male predominance, and with a very characteristic seizure semiology. The International League Against Epilepsy (ILAE) has officially renamed this syndrome as "epilepsy with myoclonic–atonic seizures."

Like other developmental epileptic encephalopathies, children with Doose syndrome have multiple seizure semiologies but the two most important are myoclonic seizures and astatic seizures (drop seizures).

Astatic seizures simply refer to a seizure causing a drop and fall. The mechanism could be variable myoclonic, negative myoclonic, or atonic. Atonic seizures are characterized by a true loss of postural tone leading to a fall. Unlike Lennox–Gastaut syndrome, children with Doose syndrome often have normal development and cognition at the onset of seizures. Also, the most common seizure semiology in Lennox–Gastaut syndrome is tonic seizures, as opposed to myoclonic seizures. Seizures can present in the presence or absence of fever. Additionally, the seizures tend to occur more commonly in the morning than at other times of day.

Around 30% of patients with Doose syndrome have a family history of seizures. Multiple gene mutations have been associated with Doose syndrome, some important ones being SLC2A1, SLC6A1, CHD2, GABRA1, SCN1A, and SCN1B. The most frequent gene mutations are SLC2A1 and SLC6A1.

Electroencephalographic evaluation may be normal at first, but most eventually develop a generalized spike-wave or polyspike-wave discharges with or without a normal background rhythm. Neuroimaging results are most often normal.

Prognosis is quite variable. Most patients achieve seizure remission in three and a half years of onset, but severe cases continue. Similarly, eventual cognitive outcome can vary from normal intellect (26–67%) to severe intellectual disability.

Commonly used anti-seizure medications include valproic acid, lamotrigine, ethosuximide, benzodiazepines, topiramate, and zonisamide. A ketogenic diet can also be used. In fact, some researchers believe that a ketogenic diet might be the most effective therapy. This is particularly true in cases caused by SLC2A1 mutation. This mutation causes GLUT-1 (glucose transporter-1) deficiency, which responds very well to a ketogenic diet.

105

• • • • •

Numb or weak, one or both legs,
Back pain, no urine stored,
Numbness in groin, all fast onset,
Compressed below the cord.

Hint #1

Try to relax and decompress. You know this.

Hint #2

Often have no "wink."

Cauda Equina Syndrome

Cauda equina syndrome (CES) is a clinically variable neurological syndrome caused by compression or distortion of the nerve roots below the spinal cord (cauda equina) prior to exiting the spinal canal. The most common cause of CES is posterior herniation of the intravertebral discs between L1 and L5, though it can also be caused by neoplasm, abscess, hematoma, or other localized swelling in the spinal canal, as well as vertebral fracture or severe spinal stenosis.

Those with CES typically present with a combination of low back and radiating pain in one or both legs, with variable degrees of weakness and/or numbness in one or both legs. These patients often also experience bowel/bladder incontinence or retention, sexual impotence in men, and decreased sensation in the perineum (saddle anesthesia). On physical exam, patients commonly have decreased or absent rectal tone, decreased or absent bulbocavernosus reflex, and decreased patellar/ankle tendon reflexes.

Besides a detailed physical exam, MRI with and without contrast of the lumbar spine (if not the complete spinal axis) is indicated to identify the compression as well as rule out other similarly presenting conditions such as transverse myelitis, multiples sclerosis, spinal cord infarction, or other myelopathies. A CT myelogram can be performed in those with contraindication to MRI, though is less sensitive.

Surgical decompression is the definitive treatment in most cases, and prognosis is dependent on both the compressive etiology and timing of successful decompression. Unfortunately, several studies have shown that regardless of the timing of decompression, approximately 50% of patients have some degree of chronic residual neurological dysfunction.

106

· · · · ·

An injured half of CNS,
Same side of body weak,
Opposite side cannot feel pain,
Same side vibration bleak.

Hint #1

Look for Horner's if at or above T1.

Hint #2

Stop halfway through.

Brown-Sequard Syndrome

Named after eccentric and controversial French physician Charles-Edouard Brown-Sequard, who first described the syndrome in 1849, Brown-Sequard syndrome (BSS) is a form of incomplete spinal cord injury. Though most often caused by acute trauma in the form of stabbing, gunshot, or severe displacing trauma to the spinal column ultimately resulting in hemi-section of the spinal cord, BSS can also be caused by more chronic progressive conditions such as spinal spondylosis, multiple sclerosis, neoplasm, radiation, or severe vertebral disc herniation. Brown-Sequard syndrome accounts for a low minority of all spinal cord injuries and has no gender predominance.

Hemi-section of the spinal cord disrupts several neuroanatomical tracts including the dorsal columns, spinothalamic tracts, ventral and dorsal spinocerebellar tracts, and the corticospinal tracts. Though symptoms vary based on the exact tracts involved, BSS is known for its characteristic sensorimotor symptoms listed below.

Ipsilateral to the Lesion

The loss of vibration, proprioception, two-point discrimination, and fine touch detection are due to injury to the ascending fibers of the dorsal columns.

Motor weakness caused by injury to the alpha motor neurons in the ventral horn presents as a lower motor neuron lesion at the level of the injury, producing decreased tone/flaccid paralysis and fasciculations, as well as upper motor neuron signs (due to injury to the corticospinal tract) below the lesion such as hypertonia, hyperreflexia, and an up-going plantar reflex.

In lesions at or above T1, injury to the descending sympathetic fibers in the intermedio-lateral column can cause ipsilateral body anhidrosis and ipsilateral ptosis and miosis (Horner's syndrome).

Contralateral to the Lesion

Loss of pain, temperature, and crude touch sensation is experienced inferior to the level of the lesion. This is because pain and temperature fibers decussate in the spinal cord and ascend as the spinothalamic tract.

Additionally, injury to the dorsal and ventral spinocerebellar tracts carrying unconscious proprioceptive sensation can cause bilateral limb ataxia to limbs below the level of the injury.

Prognosis, like in most cases of incomplete spinal cord injury, is highly variable and is based on the severity of injury and access to rehabilitation; however, overall, with rehabilitation many patients recover much of their sensory ability and strength. Most cases with structural causes will require surgical management.

107

•••••

Facial weakness on one side,
Brow weak, some hearing gain,
Treat virus/inflammation and
Few with symptoms remain.

Hint #1

Can cause hyperacusis/gustatory changes.

Hint #2

Just ask Dr. House or Dr. Brackmann.

Bell's Palsy

Named after Scottish neurologist, anatomist, and anatomical artist Sir Charles Bell following his description of the syndrome in 1821, Bell's palsy is an idiopathic peripheral facial nerve palsy (CN7) producing weakness of the unilateral upper and lower face. Though by definition, Bell's palsy is idiopathic, recent studies have proposed various viral etiologies such as the herpes simplex virus, Epstein–Barr virus, and varicella-zoster virus. In a minority of cases, the infectious causes are obvious such as in Ramsay–Hunt syndrome and Lyme disease.

The cause of the facial nerve palsy is thought to be inflammation of the facial nerve in the facial canal; more specifically, inflammation in the first portion of the facial canal, the labyrinthine segment, which is the narrowest portion.

Those with Bell's palsy typically present with one to several days of progressive unilateral facial weakness, with the peak severity of sign/symptoms being approximately three days after onset. Facial weakness can be partial or complete and often most clinically evident by decreased movement of the forehead, eyebrow, and angle of the mouth with more severe cases resulting in inability to close the eyelid. Also, because the location of facial nerve inflammation is variable, patients can also present with hyperacusis due to injury of the nerve to stapedius or gustatory changes and/or dry mouth due to injury of the chorda tympani as they branch from the facial nerve to the ear and tongue.

Evaluation of those with suspected Bell's palsy depends on the history provided by the patient. If history of tick/insect bite is reported, testing for Lyme disease is indicated. Likewise, if additional signs or symptoms are found, MRI can be useful in ruling out mimicking conditions such as schwannoma, or other compressive lesions. In those with severe cases of Bell's palsy, EMG performed several weeks after symptom onset can be helpful to determine prognosis of recovery. The severity of symptoms can be graded via the House–Brackmann severity scale.

Treatment includes eye protection in patients with incomplete eyelid closure to avoid corneal injuries. In all cases, treatment with prednisone 60 mg for seven days is recommended. In severe cases (House–Brackmann, grade IV to VI), valacyclovir is also recommended for seven days with prednisone.

Complete resolution of symptoms occurs within three to six months without treatment in the vast majority of cases (~70–85%), with a slightly greater percentage of patients reaching full recovery with treatment.

108

• • • • •

Headache after weakness one side,
Plus sensory or speech,
Spreading depression underway,
For anti-emetics reach.

Hint #1

Not a stroke, but can look like one.

Hint #2

Weakness is only temporary.

Hemiplegic Migraine

Hemiplegic migraine (HM), a rare form of migraine with aura, has a female predominance of 2–4:1 with most common onset between 12 and 17 years of age. Hemiplegic migraine can occur sporadically or pass familiarly with autosomal dominant transmission. Those with familial hemiplegic migraine (FHM) are categorized into four groups (FHM1–4) according to the gene mutation they possess. Those designated FHM1 account for approximately 50% of those with FHM and possess mutations in the CACNA1A gene on chromosome 19p13. Those with subgroups FHM2 and FMH3 possess gene mutations in ATP1A2 and SCN1A, respectively. Patients with a family history (at least one affected first-degree or second-degree relative) of HM, however, with no found gene mutation are designated FHM4.

To fulfill the diagnostic criteria for hemiplegic migraine, the presentation must first fulfill the criteria for diagnosis of migraine with aura in addition to experiencing fully reversible motor weakness, and at least one additional form of fully reversible sensory, visual, and/or speech symptoms. Though motor weakness symptoms usually resolve within 30 minutes to 72 hours, some patients report that their motor weakness persists for weeks. Making the diagnosis more difficult, hemiplegic migraine can present with or without an associated headache. Unlike the motor symptoms typical for stroke, the motor symptoms of HM often develop slowly over the course of 15–30 minutes and gradually spread along extremities (e.g., hand to arm to face). This is because of the phenomenon of cortical spreading depression, which propagates at ~3 mm/minute.

In the cases of new onset hemiplegic migraine, prolonged symptoms, and/or no family history of hemiplegic migraine, brain imaging such as non-contrasted CT or non-contrasted MRI may be indicated to rule out other conditions. Though neuroimaging is typically normal, some studies have reported meningeal enhancement and/or cerebral edema in the contralateral hemisphere to the motor symptoms. Additionally, when a reliable history is not obtainable, additional neurodiagnostic testing such as EEG or lumbar puncture may be indicated to rule out similarly presenting conditions such as Todd's paralysis, or CNS infection.

Like the treatment of migraines, treatment of HM consists of abortive therapy and preventive therapy. Generally, it is advised to avoid vasoconstrictor agents for abortive therapy because of the theoretical concern of worsening vasoconstriction. For pain symptoms, NSAIDs can be used for abortive therapy. For preventive therapy, verapamil 120 mg once daily is recommended. Alternative agents include topiramate and amitriptyline. Lamotrigine is recommended as a second-line agent. In patients with FHM, acetazolamide is recommended as treatment.

109

• • • • •

Subacute or chronic numb,
Then weakness incomplete,
Painful compression of one root,
Most common to the feet.

Hint #1

Look posterolaterally.

Hint #2

More commonly at 4 through 1.

Vertebral Disc Herniation/Radiculopathy

While back pain is the most common presenting complaint to medical clinics, herniated vertebral discs are found to be the cause in only a small minority of those cases. Herniation of vertebral discs most commonly occurs in the lumbar spine secondary to chronic degenerative changes, though not uncommonly, acute trauma can cause herniation. In either case, the intervertebral disc herniates posterolaterally onto a spinal nerve root.

The posterolateral trajectory of the herniation is due to the rigid and mostly immobile posterior longitudinal ligament that runs midline along the posterior surface of the vertebral bodies and posterior to the intervertebral disc. Herniation of the disc causes compression of the nerve root, as it leaves the spinal cord before it enters the intervertebral foramen. Because the disc usually only compresses one spinal nerve root, symptoms are most commonly experienced in one dermatomal and myotomal distribution, corresponding to the nerve root compressed (radiculopathy). Conversely, chronic spinal degenerative changes known as spondylosis can create narrowing of the spinal and intervertebral canals, producing multilevel compression of spinal nerve roots and radicular symptoms (polyradiculopathy).

The symptoms of radiculopathy are usually a combination of radiating pain from the neck (in the case of cervical radiculopathy) or low back (in the case of lumbar radiculopathy) down an extremity, with numbness and/or paresthesia felt in a dermatomal distribution. In chronic cases, patients often have decreased or absent tendon reflexes (if associated with the compromised nerve root) and the development of weakness of the associated muscles innervated by that nerve root (myotome). Regardless of acute or chronic etiology, the most common areas of vertebral disc herniation/radiculopathy are at L4 through S1 levels.

Any patient with suspected radiculopathy must undergo NCS/ EMG. This electrodiagnostic procedure will not only confirm the diagnosis but will also provide valuable information as to the severity of the radiculopathy and whether the denervation is acute or chronic.

Once the diagnosis is confirmed with NCS/EMG, MRI with and without contrast should be performed to assess for structural causes of radiculopathy such as a herniated disc.

Though not the case for herniated vertebral discs, radicular compression can have several etiologies including neoplasm, epidural hematoma, and vascular compression. All of these are best visualized and evaluated with neuroimaging using MRI. Where imaging is negative or unclear, EMG can help in evaluation and localization of symptomology.

Initial treatment usually involves conservative measures such as nonopioid pain medications and physical therapy. In some difficult cases, steroids can be used to reduce the inflammation of the compressed nerve root. For patients with significant or progressive motor deficits, surgery should be considered. In some cases of acute polyradiculopathy such as cauda equina syndrome, emergent investigation with MRI and emergent surgical decompression are indicated to prevent long-term damage.

110

• • • • •

In those with vision incomplete,
But mentally healthy,
Complex hallucinations be,
In field that they poor see.

Hint #1

Most common in those with progressive vision loss.

Hint #2

Seen much more commonly in the elderly population.

Charles Bonnet Syndrome

First described by Swiss scientist Charles Bonnet in 1760 in the case of a 90-year-old man with cataracts suffering from complex visual hallucinations in the absence of a psychiatric condition, Charles Bonnet syndrome (CBS) has become a well-known phenomenon of complex visual hallucinations in those with decreased visual acuity. Charles Bonnet syndrome can occur secondary to any disease or condition that decreases visual acuity including diabetic retinopathy, age-related macular degeneration, cerebral infarction, cataracts, glaucoma, optic ischemic or inflammatory disease, or eye trauma. The prevalence of CBS remains relatively undefined; however, it is thought to be between 0.5% and 10% of those with low visual acuity and more common in the elderly. The prevalence, however, is thought to be underestimated due to significant underreporting of visual hallucinations by the affected patient given the stigma of psychiatric illness. The most common cause of CBS is age-related visual acuity loss, particularly macular disease and glaucoma, with the most common age of symptom onset from 70 to 85 years. There is no clear male or female predominance.

Though the exact pathophysiology of CBS remains unclear, the leading theory postulates that the visual hallucinations are produced by disinhibition of cortical visual areas in the setting of decreased visual sensory input. This is thought to produce hyperactivity of the visual association regions such as the ventral occipital lobe, resulting in visual hallucinations. This is supported by the fact that CBS is not experienced by those with congenital blindness. The timing of visual hallucinations also remains unclear. However, in general, those with chronic or progressive visual acuity loss most commonly experience visual hallucinations one or more years after the onset of decreased visual acuity, while those with acute vision loss have reported visual hallucinations only days afterward.

Complex hallucinations are more common than simple hallucinations, and those with CBS often report seeing animals, creatures, or people specifically in the visual field with decreased acuity. At first these hallucinations often frighten the perceiver; however, since most patients do not have comorbid psychiatric illness, insight is often gained and the emotional response to the hallucinations decreases.

Evaluation for CBS is multidisciplinary. First the cause of decreased visual acuity should be identified through ophthalmological exam and/or neuroimaging. Additionally, the patients should be evaluated for comorbid psychiatric conditions.

Treatment is dependent on the underlying ideology of decreased visual acuity. Educating and reassuring the patient is paramount to achieving patient insight and minimizing emotional stress.

111

• • • • •

One syndrome, three lesioned parts,
In brainstem, if left be,
Left eye cannot move side to side,
Right eye just outwardly.

Hint #1

More than one but less than two.

Hint #2

Another discovery by Dr. Miller Fisher.

One and a Half Syndrome

First described by Canadian neurologist C. Miller Fisher in 1967, one and a half syndrome (OHS) is a specific pattern of ophthalmoplegia that localizes to the pons.

This syndrome is characterized by a conjugate horizontal gaze palsy toward one side with a concomitant internuclear ophthalmoparesis (INO) on attempted conjugate horizontal gaze toward the other side.

The abducens nucleus located in caudal dorso-medial pons contains interneurons and motorneurons for the lateral rectus muscle. Because of the presence of interneurons, the abducens nucleus acts as a gaze center within the pons. Descending signal from the contralateral frontal eye field, via ipsilateral superior colliculus and reticular nuclei within the paramedian pontine reticular formation (PPRF), activate the abducens nucleus. The motorneurons activate the lateral rectus muscle. The interneurons project to the contralateral medial rectus subnucleus within the oculomotor complex via MLF (medial longitudinal fasciculus).

A lesion affecting caudal dorso-medial pons can affect both the abducens nucleus and the MLF, hence producing a conjugate horizontal gaze palsy ipsilateral to the lesion and an INO with attempted conjugate gaze toward the contralateral side, hence effectively leaving only half an eye movement intact (abduction of the contralateral eye). This clinical syndrome is, hence, referred to as one and a half syndrome.

This clinical syndrome has a high localizing value. In acute settings, it warrants emergent imaging with MRI of the brain to rule out an infarction. Other common causes include pontine hemorrhage and demyelinating illness like multiple sclerosis.

Treatment will depend upon the underlying cause.

112

• • • • •

Ophthalmoplegia, painful face,
And pain behind same eye,
Not thrombosed but granulosed,
Steroids to rectify.

Hint #1

Affects 3, 4, 6, and often 5.

Hint #2

Do not let this get you *focally inflamed*.

Tolosa–Hunt Syndrome

Tolosa–Hunt syndrome (THS) was first described by Spanish neurosurgeon Edward Tolosa and later by American neurologist William E. Hunt, in 1954 and 1961, respectively, and later named after them in 1966. Tolosa–Hunt syndrome is a rare form of painful ophthalmoplegia caused by idiopathic regional inflammation of the cavernous sinus with or without associated involvement of the superior orbital fissure.

Typical presentation of THS consists of complete or partial ophthalmoplegia involving cranial nerves III (oculomotor), IV (trochlear), and VI (abducens), with periorbital or retroorbital pain and frontal or temporal headache. Additionally, in a minority of cases, facial pain in the distribution of the branches of cranial nerve V (trigeminal) as well as sympathetic involvement producing Horner's syndrome are found. Though presentation can occur at any age, the average age of presentation is in the fifth decade of life. There is no clear gender predominance. The vast majority of cases of THS are unilateral, though bilateral cases have been reported.

Tolosa–Hunt syndrome is, by definition, idiopathic; however other conditions such as trauma, tumor, and aneurysm can trigger focal inflammation, and similar presentations have been reported to be attributed to sarcoidosis, systemic, lupus erythematosus, and Wegener's granulomatosis.

Diagnostic criteria include unilateral headache and ophthalmo-legia due to the involvement of any one of the above-mentioned cranial nerves and evidence of granulomatous inflammation in the cavernous sinus as demonstrated on MRI or biopsy.

MRI with and without contrast with special focus on the cavernous sinus is essential for diagnosis. A trial of steroids with rapid improvement in symptoms within 72 hours can also be a useful diagnostic marker.

Treatment options include maintenance systemic steroids such as oral prednisone. Other options include methotrexate, azathioprine, and mycophenolate.

113

• • • • •

A lesion on one side brainstem,
Same side adduction weak,
Opposite side movements intact,
MS/infarction seek.

Hint #1

Can also see nystagmus in contralateral eye.

Hint #2

Affects the white matter tract between 3 and 6.

Internuclear Ophthalmoplegia

Internuclear ophthalmoplegia (INO) is a specific syndrome produing a characteristic ophthalmoplegia in the setting of focal lesion of the medial longitudinal fasciculus (MLF) in the brainstem. The MLF is a heavily myelinated white matter tract in the brainstem that connects various nuclei throughout the length of brainstem from medulla to midbrain. It is located in dorsal brainstem close to the midline.

To produce conjugate horizontal gaze, signal from the abducens nucleus interneurons must cross the midline via MLF and ascend to reach the medial rectus subnucleus of the oculomotor complex. A lesion of MLF on one side will disconnect the medial rectus subnucleus from the abducens nucleus interneurons on the other side, hence producing an adduction paresis on attempted conjugate horizontal gaze. A right MLF lesion will cause right adduction paresis and vice-versa.

The adduction paresis may not be complete. It is best tested by examining conjugate saccades and assessing for slow adduction movement causing the so-called adduction lag of the affected eye. In addition to the adduction paresis, the other cardinal feature of INO is the dissociated nystagmus of the abducting eye. This is not a true nystagmus though. These are saccadic oscillations. This occurs because of Hering's law of equal innervation. Because of the adduction paresis, the abducens nucleus interneurons increase innervation of the medial rectus motorneurons to overcome the deficit. But because of Hering's law, a simultaneous increase in the innervation of lateral rectus motorneurons occurs, thus causing the abducting eye to oscillate.

INO can localize anywhere in the brainstem from caudal pons to rostral midbrain. If the convergence is intact, the lesion is most likely in pons (Cogan posterior INO), but if the convergence is impaired, the lesion is most likely in the midbrain (Cogan anterior

INO). This is because of the so-called convergence center in the midbrain which is affected by a midbrain lesion as well. Other neuro-ophthalmologic findings often seen with INO include exotropia, skew deviation, and upbeat nystagmus.

Approximately one-third of cases of INO are caused by focal demyelinating disease, and an additional one-third are caused by brainstem infarction. Treatment depends on the underlying cause. If the diplopia is severe, patching of one eye can be done.

114

• • • • •

Sense of movement room within,
A crystal out of place,
Torsional nystagmus seen,
If laid supine, side face.

Benign Paroxysmal Positional Vertigo (BPPV)

First described in German by Dr. D. Adler (unknown first name) in 1897 as the "one-sided rotary vertigo," then later by Austrian otologist Robert Barany in 1921, benign paroxysmal positional vertigo (BPPV) finally received its name from Margaret Dix and Charles Hallpike in 1952.

Benign paroxysmal positional vertigo is an inducible, transient illusion of environmental motion, producing nausea, imbalance, and rotatory or torsional nystagmus. This is caused by dislodged and free-floating otoliths, which are crystalline structures made of calcium carbonate, normally embedded in the otolithic membranes of the macula of both the utricle and saccule of the inner ear that, once dislodged from the otolithic membrane, travel through the semicircular canals producing distortions in endolymph movement and ultimately the illusory perception of movement. From the Greek words *oto-* (ear) and *lithos* (stones), otoliths are a normal anatomical microstructure of the inner ear that aid with the perception of head motion in all planes of movement.

The most common age of onset for BPPV is 50–70 years old with a slight female predominance. Most cases of BPPV are idiopathic and thought to be due to age-related otolithic membrane degeneration. A minority of cases are considered secondary BPPV and result from other causes such as head trauma or inner ear surgery.

Patients with BPPV most often present with episodic vertigo. These episodes are triggered by the rotation of the head against gravity, for example, rolling over in bed. Episodes often produce severe imbalance, nausea, and sometimes vomiting, but commonly resolve spontaneously within 60 seconds.

Diagnosis is made both by patient history and by redemonstration of the symptoms using the Dix–Hallpike maneuver. This maneuver quickly takes the patient from sitting to laying supine with their head rotated 45 degrees to one side, hanging at the edge of the bed. Here the head is held motionless for 30 seconds as the patient's eyes are watched for the nystagmus, and the patient is questioned about the reemergence of their typical vertiginous symptoms. Depending on the type of nystagmus seen and symptom reemergence, as well as the utilization of other symptom eliciting maneuvers, a diagnosis of either posterior canal BPPV (most common), lateral canal BPPV, or anterior canal BPPV (least common) can be made.

Treatment can include one of several available particle-repositioning maneuvers, depending on the type of BPPV the patient is suspected of having, as well as the physical capabilities of the patient and provider. The most commonly used maneuver is the modified Epley maneuver for posterior canal BPPV.

115

• • • • •

Acute in onset vertigo,
Post-viral symptoms glean,
Contralateral fast phase,
An inflamed nerve is seen.

Hint #1

Notably no hearing loss.

Hint #2

Resolves spontaneously.

Vestibular Neuritis/Vestibular Neuronitis

Caused by inflammation of the vestibular portion of cranial nerve eight (vestibulocochlear nerve), vestibular neuritis (VN) is one of the most common causes of acute peripheral vertigo. Though the exact cause of highly localized inflammation is unknown, it is generally thought to be caused by post-viral inflammation, especially to latent HSV.

Vestibular neuritis presents as acute vestibular syndrome. This clinical syndrome is defined by acute onset persistent vertigo, which is not dependent on head position. It is associated with profound nausea and vomiting. There are two major differential diagnoses for acute vestibular syndrome – vestibular neuritis and stroke. The distinction can be made by clinical examination.

The nystagmus in VN is a mixed horizontal–torsional nystagmus with the fast phase beating away from the affected ear. The nystagmus increases in amplitude when looking toward the direction of the fast phase (Alexander's law). There is no skew deviation. With the head impulse test from the affected side, the fixation breaks, and a catch-up saccade can be seen (positive head impulse test).

The nystagmus with central causes such as brainstem stroke is usually purely torsional or vertical (upbeat or downbeat). This is often associated with a skew deviation as well, which refers to a vertical misalignment. The head impulse test is negative.

This combination of examination maneuvers is referred to as HINTS (head impulse, nystagmus, skew). This constellation of exam findings is more sensitive than a brain MRI in distinguishing VN from a brainstem stroke.

Unlike the episodic nature of the symptoms experienced in BPPV, the symptoms of VN are persistent, develop over hours, usually reaching their worst between day one and two. Approximately half of patients report a viral illness prodrome or concurrent viral illness symptoms. Most cases of VN will resolve spontaneously within one week of symptom onset.

Treatment of VN mainly consists of symptomatic management with a single or combination of short-term antiemetics, antihistamines, and benzodiazepines. Most studies testing treatment with corticosteroids and/or antiviral medications have reported insufficient proof of their efficacy.

116

• • • • •

Chang'ed gene within, this condition,
Nerve two has tumors through,
Iris and skin with changed pigment in,
Of nerves fibromas grew.

Hint #1

Tumor growth is usually benign.

Hint #2

While you think, have a French coffee with milk.

Neurofibromatosis Type 1

First called von Recklinghausen disease, named after German pathologist Friedrich Daniel von Recklinghausen in 1882, neurofibromatosis type 1 (NF1) is a genetic neurocutaneous condition, making up 96% of all cases of neurofibromatosis. With a loss of function mutation (50% are inherited, 50% de novo) of the neurofibromin 1 gene on chromosome 11, those with NF1 have nonfunctional neurofibromin, which functions in the mTOR and RAS/MAPK pathways as a tumor suppressor. Neurofibromatosis type 1 has an autosomal dominant inheritance pattern and has no gender predominance.

The clinical manifestations of NF1 are highly variable, but most commonly first presents prepubertally with multiple small (5–15 mm) sharply demarcated tan-brown café-au-lait (from French, meaning "coffee with milk") macules as well as groin and axillary freckling. In the peripubertal years, neurofibromas appear, which can be cutaneous, appearing as flesh-colored, dome-shaped soft skin growths, or internal, which are derived from nerve sheaths and felt under the skin as a "bag of worms." Though cutaneous neurofibromas are benign, internal neurofibromas, known as plexiform neurofibromas have a 5–15% chance of becoming malignant in adulthood. Approximately 90% of those with NF1 have benign iris hamartomas (Lisch nodules) by age 20, which appear as 1–2 mm-sized yellow-brown papules. Also, optic gliomas can be seen in ~15% of children with NF1.

Though in general no treatment is needed for café-au-lait spots or cutaneous neurofibromas, clinical monitoring for malignant transformation of plexiform neurofibromas is indicated in cases where they rapidly increase in size or become hard or the patients develop localized pain or exihibit neurological deficits.

117

· · · · ·

In young, seizures, and with nodules,
In ventricles they line,
Fibrous plaques in brain and eye,
With skin changes benign.

Hint #1

Commonly presents early with seizures.

Hint #2

Blame it on hamartin and tuberin.

Tuberous Sclerosis

Tuberous sclerosis (TS) is a genetic neurocutaneous syndrome caused by either sporadic (most common) or autosomal dominant inheritance of a mutation of the TSC1 (chromosome 9) or TSC2 (chromosome 16) genes. These genes encode for the proteins hamartin and tuberin, respectively, which are negative regulators of the mTOR pathway.

Clinically, the signs and symptoms of TS start in early childhood and become disabling through the patient's lifetime. The neurological features of TS include the formation of benign cortical hamartomas, called tubers, which are found in 95% of those with TS and thought to be responsible for the associated early childhood epilepsy these patients develop. Those with TS also commonly have subependymal nodules, which are hamartomatous growths that often calcify as well as degenerate to subependymal giant cell astrocytomas (SEGAs). Though SEGAs grow very slowly, they can cause obstructive hydrocephalus. These cerebral manifestations ultimately cause seizures and intellectual delay in most patients.

Cutaneous manifestations of TS include areas of hypopigmented skin lesions known as "ash leaf macules" as well as "confetti hypopigmentation," which appear as much smaller lighter skin spots scattered around the ash leaf macule. Also, those with TS also have "Shagreen patches," which are slightly larger plaques of connective tissue nevus that can vary in pigmentation. Renal angiomyolipomas, cardiac rhabdomyomas, and retinal astrocytic hamartomas are the other common clinical features of TS.

Most patients with TS develop refractory epilepsy. West syndrome is a type of early childhood onset developmental epileptic encephalopathy characterized by epileptic spasms, developmental delay, and interictal EEG finding of hypsarrhythmia. The most common cause of West syndrome is TS. The usual line of treatment for West syndrome is ACTH. Vigabatrin is preferred over ACTH in TS.

Periodic brain MRIs once every one to three years are recommended for TS patients, up to the age of 25, to watch for the progression of SEGAs. Initial echocardiogram is also recommended to screen for rhabdomyomas. Frequent renal MRIs are recommended to monitor the progression of renal angiomyolipomas.

Everolimus, which is an mTOR pathway inhibitor, has been shown to reduce seizure frequency and is also used for the treatment of angiofibromas and renal angiomyolipomas.

118

• • • • •

Sense of movement, ears are ringing,
Hearing becomes less,
Reducing increased endolymph,
Lessens sense of fullness.

Hint #1

Episodes not triggered by head motion.

Hint #2

Think inner ear dilation.

Ménière Disease

Ménière disease (MD) is a relatively rare disorder of the inner ear classically producing the triad of hearing loss, vertigo, and either tinnitus or a sense of ear fullness with most common onset between 50 and 70 years of age and slight female predominance. Also known as idiopathic endolymphatic hydrops, MD is named after French physician Prosper Ménière after his linking of the condition to the inner ear in 1861. Though the exact pathophysiology remains unclear, MD appears to either be caused by or associated with endolymphatic accumulation in organs of the inner ear, namely, the cochlea, semicircular canals, ampulla, and saccule. Dysfunction is thought to be due to the compensatory dilation of the endolymphatic spaces and caused by unequal endolymph secretion and reabsorption.

Clinically, these patients often present with spontaneous recurrent vertigo lasting more than 20 minutes but less than 12 hours. Of note, unlike benign paroxysmal positional vertigo, vertiginous attacks in MD are typically not triggered by rotation of the head. Hearing loss is most commonly unilateral, but can become bilateral, progressive but with fluctuation, and affecting primary low–medium frequency audition. The tinnitus and/or sense of "ear fullness" reported by those with MD is usually experienced in the same ear as the one with hearing loss.

Audiometric testing is recommended. It often shows low to mid frequency sensorineural hearing loss.

Initial management consists of lifestyle changes including decreasing salt intake and limiting coffee and alcohol intake as well. Vestibular rehabilitation is also recommended. For chronic management, medications like betahistine and diuretics are often used. For patients with refractory symptoms, systemic steroids or intratympanic steroids are used. Rarely for super-refractory cases, surgical procedures such as labyrinthectomy or vestibular neurectomy can be performed.

119

• • • • •

Most patients with psych history,
Withdrawn or agitated,
Limbs stay where put, phrases repeat,
Till benzo medicated.

Hint #1

Do not know, ask Bush-Francis.

Hint #2

Often unresponsive.

Catatonia

Catatonia, first categorized as its own entity in 1874 by Karl Kahlbaum, is a psychomotor syndrome broadly characterized by a lack of communication and abnormal movement. Though catatonia is commonly associated with several mental health disorders such as schizophrenia, mania, and bipolar disorder, it has also been reported in the cases of hyponatremia, Parkinson disease, cerebral infarction or neoplasm, and benzodiazepine withdrawal.

According to the DSM-5, diagnosis of catatonia requires the presence of ≥3 of the following: mutism, abnormal posturing, waxy flexibility, stupor, catalepsy, stereotypies, grimacing, agitation, negativism, echopraxia, and echolalia. There are a few clinical scales that help diagnose and determine the severity of catatonia including the Bush-Francis catatonia rating scale and the Northoff catatonia scale.

According to the general symptomatic presentation of those with catatonia, they are grouped into the subtypes akinetic catatonia, excited catatonia, and malignant catatonia. Broadly characterizing, those with akinetic catatonia present with staring and either unresponsiveness or hyporesponsiveness to verbal or tactile stimuli, though are aware of their surroundings. Those with excited catatonia generally have impulsive and purposeless movements and often appear to be agitated or even combative. Malignant catatonia can be life-threatening and is associated with dysfunction of the autonomic nervous system such as dangerous variations in blood pressure, heart rate, temperature, and respiratory rate, and sometimes appear diaphoretic.

The diagnosis of catatonia is usually confirmed by the lorazepam challenge test. Intravenous lorazepam 1 mg or 2 mg dose is administered, and the patient is observed for temporary improvement of symptoms within 5–10 minutes to confirm the diagnosis.

Malignant catatonia can be life-threatening and hence must be treated emergently. Immediate treatment of the underlying disorder (psychiatric or medical) must be initiated along with electroconvulsive therapy. For nonmalignant catatonia, the treatment for the underlying cause must be initiated. If there is no response within one week, electroconvulsive therapy can be considered. For patients who do not want to pursue electroconvulsive therapy, other medical options include topiramate, carbamazepine, and amantadine.

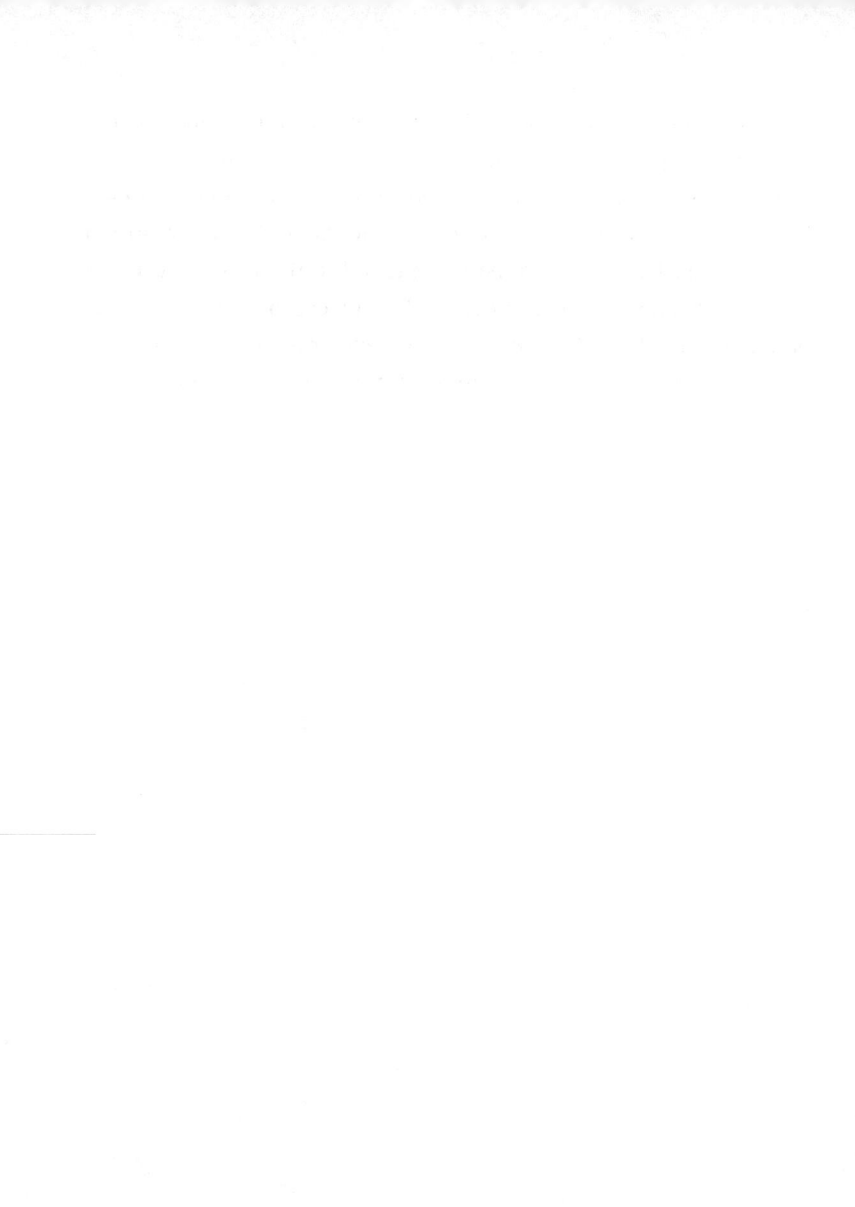

120

• • • • •

Over hours both legs weak,
Back pain, no wink, legs numb
No trauma, or effacement seen,
But restriction sure to come.

Hint #1

Either anterior or posterior.

Hint #2

Look out for aortic disease.

Spinal Cord Infarction (Anterior Spinal Artery Occlusion)

First described in 1904 in the case of an anterior spinal artery occlusion, spinal cord infarction is a devastating neurological condition constituting approximately only 1% of CNS infarctions. Though data on the frequency and etiology of spinal cord infarction is limited, most cases occur spontaneously in the setting of aortic arteriosclerosis or perioperatively and associated with aortic procedure.

The majority of spinal cord infarctions occur from occlusion of the anterior spinal artery and more commonly at the level of the thoracolumbar spinal cord segments rather than the cervical cord. Unlike cerebral infarctions, signs of spinal cord infarction often develop over hours.

Because the spinal cord receives dual blood supply from the anterior spinal artery and the posterior spinal artery, infarction does not affect all spinal cord tracts and can be grouped accordingly into anterior spinal cord syndrome and posterior spinal cord syndrome. Patients with anterior spinal cord syndrome, caused by occlusion of the anterior spinal artery, present with acute symptoms of back pain, paraplegia, or tetraplegia, hypoesthesia or anesthesia to pain and temperature in the bilateral affected limbs, as well as bowel and bladder dysfunction. Anal wink is usually absent in acute spinal cord infarction. Those with posterior spinal cord syndrome, caused by occlusion of the posterior spinal artery, often present with acute symptoms of back pain (though less commonly than in anterior spinal artery occlusion), as well as loss of vibration and proprioceptive sense. Given high variability in spinal perfusion, up to 50% of those with an otherwise anterior spinal artery territory infarction can present with some degree of proprioceptive deficit.

The diagnosis is mainly clinical, but a spinal MRI is required to mainly rule out compressive etiologies. T2 sequences can show a hyperintensity within the spinal cord but the diffusion-weighted images have higher sensitivity.

Treatment is mainly supportive. There is not enough evidence to suggest the use of thrombolytics. Spinal cord ischemia remains a dreaded complication of thoracic endovascular aortic repair (TEVAR). Patients who are at high risk include those who have had a previous surgery or have had a prior aortic dissection. Those with the procedure being done between T6 and L2 levels are also at high risk, since this is the level where the artery of Adamkiewicz reinforces the anterior spinal artery. Such patients should have a lumbar drain placed intraoperatively and should be monitored using intraoperative neurophysiology with somatosensory and motor evoked potentials.

If signs and symptoms of spinal cord ischemia develop post-op, the mean arterial pressure should be increased by 10mmHg every 5 minutes until symptoms resolve. If symptoms do not improve within 10 minutes, lumbar drain must be placed if not already in place.

Overall, up to 46% of patients can achieve ambulatory status while up to 57% do not. A lack of improvement within the first 24 hours is a poor prognostic sign.

121

• • • • •

Hypersexuality,
Amnesia, hyperoral,
Hypermetamorphosis,
Lesions in both temporal.

Hint #1

No weakness or somatosensory loss.

Hint #2

Not a primary psychiatric condition.

Kluver–Bucy Syndrome

First described in 1888 by neurologists Schafer and Brown, and later in 1939 by German American experimental psychologist Heinrick Kluver and American neurosurgeon Paul Clancy Bucy, now named Kluver–Bucy syndrome (KBS), this condition was first described after bilateral temporal lobectomy in monkeys. It was later described in humans in 1955 in the case of a 19-year-old male with epilepsy, again requiring treatment with bilateral temporal lobectomy.

Today, KBS is known as a rare neuropsychiatric disorder caused by injury to the bilateral amygdalae. Given bilateral temporal lobectomies are no longer performed in humans, modern cases of KBS are most commonly caused by severe brain trauma, neurodegenerative disease, and cerebral infections such as herpes simplex virus encephalitis. Because of the complex structure and function of the temporal lobes, the exact mechanism of the KBS is unknown, though thought to be due to the disruption of the limbic network, ultimately causing disinhibition, changes in affect, and emotional regulation. These changes include hypersexuality (with both animate and inanimate objects), hyperorality (compulsive licking or placing objects in mouth), binging and purging eating behavior, hypermetamorphosis (the impulse to notice and react to all things in sight), visual agnosia, and flat affect.

Because KBS is caused by structural dysfunction of the bilateral temporal lobe structures, treatment is difficult and focuses on symptom management.

122

• • • • •

In patients high in A1C,
Get asymmetric pain,
In hips then proximal weakness,
Then waste, then symptoms wane.

Hint #1

Self-limiting.

Hint #2

Usually in well-controlled patients.

Diabetic Amyotrophy

Also known as diabetic lumbosacral radiculoplexus neuropathy, Bruns–Garland syndrome, and many other names, diabetic amyotrophy (DA) is an uncommon (~1% of those with diabetes) and clinically variable asymmetric diabetic neuropathy with unclear pathophysiology. It is generally thought that DA is an immune-mediated microvasculitis causing ischemic nerve injury involving the lumbosacral plexus, nerve roots, and peripheral nerves.

Though the vast majority of patients with DA have type II diabetes, it can present in those with type-1 diabetes, and most of them also have good glycemic control. Diabetic amyotrophy also has a predominance in men above the age of 50.

The clinical presentation is overall relatively consistent between cases, and usually consists of an episodic, monophasic, acute to subacute asymmetric syndrome of unilateral proximal lower extremity pain (usually the first symptoms), and proximal hip and thigh muscle weakness, followed by the atrophy of the affected muscles and associated weight loss. These patients often also have some components of sensory loss and areflexia in the affected leg, and can present with autonomic nervous system dysfunction, most commonly orthostatic hypotension. Notably, though these patients most often present with asymmetric symptoms, some degree of pain and weakness is usually present bilaterally at some point during the course of DA; however, it usually occurs after several months of unilateral symptom progression.

Nerve conduction studies with needle electromyography are part of the routine diagnostic investigation. MRI lumbar spine and lumbosacral plexus with and without contrast is also recommended to evaluate for inflammation of the nerve roots and the peripheral nerves within the plexus. This also helps to rule out other causes of a similar clinical syndrome.

DA is a self-limiting condition, and symptoms often begin to subside after one year, first with improvement in pain, then in strength. Only a minority of those with DA will have residual weakness or pain after two years. Treatment is mainly symptomatic aimed at the pain. Commonly used medications include selective serotonin reuptake inhibitors (SSRIs), serotonin-nerepinephrine reuptake inhibitors (SNRIs), and gabapentin/pregabalin. Physical and occupational therapy are recommended for the improvement of weakness.

123

• • • • •

In malnourished, B is low,
Dementia onset fast or slow,
Hemispheres show disconnect,
Lesioned corpus will then show.

Hint #1

Focal demyelination.

Hint #2

Some improved with nutritional supplementation.

Marchiafava–Bignami Disease (Degeneration of the Corpus Collosum)

First described by Italian pathologists Ettore Marchiafava and Amico Bignami in 1903, Marchiafava–Bignami disease (MBD) is a degenerative disease localized primarily to the heavily myelinated tracts of the corpus collosum.

Though MBD was originally thought to be caused by the toxic effects of alcohol, it has been reported in those abstinent of alcohol, thus raising concern that it may be due to a nutritional deficiency. Interestingly, however, no causal deficiency has been identified, though some cases report improvement with thiamine supplementation. The neurophysiology and neuropathology of MBD are also somewhat of a mystery as these patients have demyelination and noninflammatory necrosis of the white matter that is almost completely selective to the corpus collosum. Rarely, however, this can also be found symmetrically in nearby white matter such as the superior cerebellar peduncles or centrum semiovale.

The vast majority of cases of MBD have been found in men in mid to late adulthood with alcoholism. Unfortunately, there is no symptomatic syndrome that is consistent in those with MBD, as signs and symptoms vary widely in reported cases, from stupor and coma to alert with seizures, tremors, and hallucinations (delirium tremens), to progressive dementia. Some degree of improvement has been reported in several cases after nutritional restoration.

124

• • • • •

In children oft' with tumor that,
Immune system tries to combat,
Eyes and feet will jerk and dance,
And need support with talk/with stance.

Hint #1

Also found in adults with cancer.

Hint #2

Think peripheral neuroblastoma.

Opsoclonus–Myoclonus–Ataxia Syndrome

Also called opsoclonus–myoclonus syndrome or dancing eye-dancing feet syndrome, opsoclonus–myoclonus-ataxia syndrome (OMAS) is a rare paraneoplastic movement disorder, on the spectrum of childhood-acquired cerebellar ataxias, which typically presents in children <5 years old with neuroblastoma.

In approximately 50% of children with OMAS, a co-occurring early-stage peripheral neuroblastic tumor is found, with neuroblastoma being the most commonly found, followed by ganglioneuroblastoma and ganglioneuroma, respectively. These tumors are always extracranial and are typically found in the sympathetic chain or adrenal glands. Contrary to the paraneoplastic etiology hypothesis, a minority of these patients do not exhibit a neoplastic process. Unfortunately, there have been no consistently found biomarkers linking OMAS to any paraneoplastic process.

Children with OMAS can present first with either ataxia, myoclonus, or opsoclonus. Opsoclonus is characterized by saccadic intrusions without intersaccadic interval in multiple directions. These patients also often have some degree of behavior changes such as irritability and sleep disturbance, which along with balance difficulties can result in temporary regression of motor and language skills. Interestingly, OMAS is also found in adults with breast cancer and small cell lung cancer.

Any child presenting with OMAS must undergo thorough evaluation for neuroblastoma. If neuroblastoma is detected, then treatment of neuroblastoma must be initiated immediately along with the treatment for OMAS. OMAS is usually treated with a combination of IVIG and steroids. Other treatment options include rituximab and cyclophosphamide.

In adults with paraneoplastic OMAS, the most frequent cancer is small cell lung cancer. An extensive search to detect cancer must be performed in adults presenting with OMAS. A specific antibody may not be found.

125

• • • • •

Bilateral lesions in back,
Occip-parietal,
Cannot reach objects/turn eyes to see,
Sees only one when dual.

Hint #1

A famous triad of symptoms.

Hint #2

Cannot see the forest for the trees.

Balint Syndrome

First described by Hungarian neurologist Rezso Balint in 1909 and initially called "triple-complex syndrome," Balint syndrome (later named after him in 1954) is a triad of symptoms involving attention and coordination of voluntary eye movements in patients with bilateral parieto-occipital lobe lesions. Though published reports of Balint syndrome have almost all been in case report form, and epidemiological trends cannot be generalized, cases have been reported in many conditions including but not limited to cerebral infarction, hemorrhage, neurodegenerative disease, posterior reversible encephalopathy syndrome, brain trauma, brain tumor, CNS infection, autoimmune encephalitis, and prion disease.

Balint syndrome is known for its unique triad of symptoms including simultanagnosia, optic ataxia, and oculomotor apraxia. Simultanagnosia is a form of visual attention deficit with the inability to see more than one object at a time. For example, if a patient is shown a picture of a garden, they might only see a flower, and might be unable to pay simultaneous visual attention to the picture of the garden as a whole of its parts.

Optic ataxia is characterized by the inability to reach out and grab an object that the patient can see and is within reach. Oculomotor apraxia is the inability to generate voluntary saccades. Patients often make head thrusts to move their eyes in the desired direction. Visual cue-based smooth pursuit movements are intact.

Diagnosis is based on the presence of these three cardinal signs and bilateral parieto-occipital lesions on neuroimaging. Treatment is based on the underlying etiology, with prognosis varying widely based on that etiology.

126

• • • • •

Sudden onset pain then weak,
In shoulder, then resolved,
Post-infection or immune,
Denervated nerves involved.

Hint #1

Many with viral prodrome weeks before.

Hint #2

Also seen after radiation treatment.

Parsonage–Turner Syndrome/Brachial Plexitis

Known by many names including brachial plexitis, brachial plexus neuritis, brachial neuritis, and neuralgic amyotrophy, Parsonage–Turner syndrome (PTS) was first well described by British neurologists M.J. Parsonage and John Turner in *The Lancet* in 1948. They described "a syndrome of pain and flaccid paralysis of the muscles around the shoulder joint" in 136 patients and remarked on the high incidence of factors preceding the symptoms, of which most patients were found to have a precipitating infection (71), surgical procedure or medical treatment (17), or trauma (10). Though we know more about PTS today, these trends remain overall consistent.

Most cases of PTS are diagnosed in those who are 20–60 years old, and twice as often in men than in women. Though the etiology remains uncertain, modern cases appear to be precipitated by viral infection or vaccination in 25% and 15%, respectively, leading researchers to suspect either an autoimmune or direct viral cause.

The clinical presentation of PTS most often appears one to four weeks after an immunological stressor with a unilateral acute aching pain in the superolateral shoulder that is nonpositional and usually worse at night. These painful symptoms often resolve spontaneously over days to several weeks, then followed by painless mainly proximal weakness in the same shoulder and arm, most commonly affecting shoulder abduction and external rotation. Atrophy of the shoulder muscles can be seen. Strength often returns after 6–18 months. Paresthesias or hypoesthesia of the shoulder and lateral arm is common.

Diagnosis is mainly clinical. Nerve conduction studies with needle electromyography are usually performed. These studies demonstrate the presence of active denervation. There is no specific treatment. Pain management and physical therapy are recommended.

127

• • • • •

Sudden intermittent weak,
If carbs post-exercise,
Channelopathy within,
Low mineral in lies.

Hint #1

Mainly thought of as hereditary.

Hint #2

Primarily in limbs, not respiratory/bulbar.

Hypokalemic Periodic Paralysis

Hypokalemic periodic paralysis (HPP) is a rare hereditary or acquired condition resulting in episodes of severe muscle weakness, usually in the setting of strenuous exercise with a high carbohydrate diet. The most common form of HPP is inherited (familial hypokalemic periodic paralysis) and is caused by either a mutation in the skeletal muscle calcium channel gene CACNA1S (HPP type 1) or the skeletal muscle sodium channel gene SCN4A (HPP type 2). Thyrotoxicosis can also cause HPP (acquired HPP). Familial HPP follows an autosomal dominant inheritance pattern and exhibits incomplete penetrance, with a male predominance. Though ~80% of cases of familial HPP are caused by CACNA1S, SCN4A, or KCNJ2 gene mutations, the genetic cause of the rest remains undetermined.

Most cases of HPP present for the first time in late childhood or during teenage years with the exception of thyrotoxic HPP, which first presents after 20 years of age. The most common presentation is triggered by strenuous exercise or after a large carbohydrate meal. After this meal, it is thought that insulin increases and serum potassium drops as potassium shifts intracellularly, which causes the episode of weakness. There is usually a lag of hours between the trigger and the onset of paralysis.

Though some patients report experiencing a prodrome of paresthesias or fatigue, most patients report waking up the day after strenuous exercise with their symptoms of profound proximal more than distal limb weakness, most prominent in the lower extremities. Reflexes are typically decreased. The frequency and severity of weakness episodes vary widely in patients, ranging from minutes to several days prior to resolution.

Thyroid function test with TSH, free T3 and T4 must be performed to rule out thyrotoxicosis as an acquired cause of PP. Electrolytes, especially potassium levels must be checked during the attack and in between attacks to demonstrate normal potassium levels. Genetic testing can be performed to identify the underlying mutation.

An electrodiagnostic procedure called long exercise test (LET) is often performed to diagnose any form of PP, including hypokalemic PP. This consists of recording a baseline CMAP, followed by sequential recording every 1–2 minutes after 4–5 minutes of exercise. After about 30–40 minutes of testing, a decline of CMAP amplitude by more than 40% is suggestive of PP.

Patients with hypokalemic PP must also undergo an electrocardiogram to evaluate for prolonged QT interval to diagnose Andersen-Tawil syndrome. These patients are at high risk of ventricular arrhythmias and sudden cardiac death.

Treatment during acute attacks requires gradual replacement of potassium. Preventive treatment involves avoiding known triggers. Medications such as acetazolamide and spironolactone can also be used.

128

• • • • •

Mydriasis in dark and light,
When look near will slow contract,
Tendon reflexes decreased,
Ciliary not intact.

Hint #1

Exhibit light-near dissociation.

Hint #2

Big pupil will however constrict with pilocarpine.

Holmes–Adie Syndrome

Named after British neurologist William Adie and Irish neurologist Sir Gordon Holmes after first describing the condition (calling it "pseudo-Argyll Robertson pupil" in 1931), Holmes–Adie syndrome (HAS) is characterized by pupillary dysfunction and areflexia. Though the exact cause is unclear, HAS appears to involve the degeneration of the ciliary ganglion resulting in postganglionic parasympathetic fiber impairment and ultimately dysfunction of the pupil. Most cases of HAS are idiopathic; however, cases have been linked to systemic infection (mainly viral), autoimmune diseases including paraneoplastic conditions and other systemic inflammatory diseases, orbital tumors and local trauma, and neuromuscular conditions, among many other published causes.

Those with HAS present with mydriasis of the affected eye and often complain of blurry vision or photophobia. On exam, the affected pupil does not constrict or minimally constricts in response to direct light. Characteristic to HAS, these patients exhibit light-near dissociation meaning just like in the condition of Argyll Robertson pupil, the affected pupil will constrict with near vision (accommodation) but not with direct light. Interestingly, once the affected pupil is constricted, it remains constricted for an extended time (tonic pupil) and returns to its normal dilated state slowly. Helpful in diagnosis, HAS is highly responsive to miotic drugs such as pilocarpine. Those with HAS can also exhibit segmental pupillary sphincter palsy and appear to have an irregular pupil shape.

Most patients do not usually require any treatment. This is considered a benign condition and patients usually just require reassurance.

129

• • • • •

Sudden negative symptoms,
In minutes oft resolved,
ABCD2 to score,
Once the issue has dissolved.

Hint #1

Not always embolic.

Hint #2

Look out for impending stroke.

Transient Ischemic Attack

Transient ischemic attacks (TIAs) are characterized as transient focal neurological episodes, usually lasting only minutes, which correspond with a vascular territory and resolve spontaneously leaving no permanent clinical sign or observable changes on neuroimaging. These episodes can theoretically involve any cerebrovascular territory. The mechanism behind TIAs is thought to be either hypoperfusion of a vascular territory due to reduced blood flow in the setting of focal vascular stenosis or an embolic particle that dissolves shortly after occluding a vessel.

Because any cerebrovascular territory can be involved, those with a TIA often present with sudden unilateral hemiparesis, unilateral numbness, aphasia, dysarthria, ataxia, visual field blindness, diplopia, or a combination that would represent a known stroke syndrome. Interestingly, there have been reports of TIAs producing positive symptoms as well, including tingling paresthesias and even limb shaking.

The higher risk demographics for TIA are generally the same as for cerebral infarction and include an older male predominance, with a history of tobacco use, hypertension, hyperlipidemia, diabetes, and previous cerebrovascular events. Because of their vascular mechanism, TIAs are also a significant risk factor for the occurrence of future ischemic stroke, with 20% of those with TIA experiencing an ischemic stroke within one month of the event, and 50% within a year of the event. Because of the significant risk of future ischemic stroke, a rapid clinical assessment focused on the patient's demographics and symptoms was developed called the ABCD2 score.

Age: ≥ 60 years (1 point)
Blood pressure: on presentation ≥140/90 mmHg (1 point)

Clinical symptoms:

   –focal weakness (2 points)

   –or speech impairment without weakness (1 point)

Duration: $\geq$ 60 min (2 points) or 10 min to 59 min (1 point)

Diabetes mellitus: (1 point)

The diagnosis of TIA is made clinically and primarily focuses on obtaining an accurate characteristic history of the event and confirmation of no infarction on neuroimaging (MRI is needed to evaluate for acute infarction). The treatment of a TIA focuses on risk factor minimization.

130

• • • • •

Increased heart rate upon rising,
Light headed, toe color change,
Many with small fiber problem,
Blood pressure remains normal range.

Hint #1

A form of dysautonomia.

Hint #2

In the absence of orthostatic hypotension.

Postural Orthostatic Tachycardia Syndrome

Postural orthostatic tachycardia syndrome (POTS) is a form of dysautonomia generally characterized as a disproportionate tachycardia and orthostatic intolerance upon standing. Though the prevalence of POTS is unknown, there is a significant predominance in premenstrual Caucasian females with the highest rate of first presentation between 15 and 25 years of age. The pathophysiology of POTS is unknown; however, it is thought to be a combination of multiple dysfunctional comorbidities such as impaired intravascular volume regulation, cardiac deconditioning, peripheral autonomic neuropathy, and increased sympathetic tone, which in combination can create an exaggerated sympathetic response to standing.

To date, there is no consensus on a unified etiology for POTS; however, there are several proposed theories, which have led to the proposal of multiple possible POTS subtypes.

- The so-called hyperadrenergic POTS subtype is characterized by elevated plasma norepinephrine concentration in combination with other signs of increased sympathetic drive such as tachycardia, tremor, hypertension, palpitations, and anxiety.
- Another subtype is neuropathic POTS that postulates POTS as a length-dependent autonomic neuropathy, resulting in reduced venous constriction and subsequent venous pooling in the lower extremities requiring an excessive cardiovascular response to maintain optimal arterial pressures when standing.
- In hypovolemic POTS subtype, it is proposed that low plasma/total blood volume in the setting of low renin and angiotensin levels is caused by the dysfunction of the renin–angiotensin–aldosterone axis, ultimately causing low intravascular volume.
- Others propose that POTS is secondary to deconditioning or is associated with an autoimmune condition given its female

predominance, viral illness prodrome, and higher proportion of patients with elevated autoimmune markers such as anti-nuclear antibodies and IL6.

The diagnostic criteria for POTS requires only an increase in heart rate of ≥30 bpm within 10 minutes after standing or after a head-up tilt table test (the gold standard for assessment) in the absence of orthostatic hypotension. Patients with POTS often also present with complaints of palpitations, lightheadedness, fatigue, abdominal/suprapubic pain, nausea, Raynaud's phenomenon, and cognitive impairment.

The management of POTS involves lifestyle measures such as increasing salt intake and maintaining adequate hydration. Compressive stockings and abdominal binders can be used in difficult cases. For refractory cases, pharmacologic treatment can be used. Beta blockers such as propranolol can be effective. Other options include midodrine and fludrocortisone.

131

· · · · ·

Sudden headache, narrowed vessels,
Post-part/SSRI,
Some with stroke but no clot in,
For most symptoms go bye.

Hint #1

Need some help? Call-Fleming.

Hint #2

One cause of thunderclap headache.

Reversible Cerebral Vasoconstriction Syndrome

Reversible cerebral vasoconstriction syndrome (RCVS), previously called benign angiopathy of the central nervous system, call-Fleming syndrome, or migrainous vasospasm, is a form of transient multifocal arterial vasospasm and vasodilation. The exact pathophysiology of RCVS is unknown; however, it is thought to be due to a temporary dysregulation of cerebrovascular tone.

Though some cases of RCVS are idiopathic, most have suspected triggers such as vasoactive medications including sympathomimetic and migraine medication and illegal recreational drugs. Additionally, several medical conditions have been associated with increased risk of developing RCVS such as systemic autoimmune conditions, recent head or neck trauma/procedure, and early postpartum state.

Most patients with RCVS are female (2–3:1) and are between 20 and 50 years of age. They present with recurrent severe sudden onset worst headache of their life (thunderclap headache) with maximum intensity within seconds to minutes. These patients also often have co-occurring confusion, vomiting, blurry vision, and in severe cases seizure and focal weakness or numbness.

The diagnosis is mainly clinically based on a high degree of suspicion. An initial MRI may be completely normal. Some typical findings include multifocal small infarcts and sulcal subarachnoid hemorrhages. A CT angiogram or an MR angiogram must also be performed to assess for vasospasm. Multifocal vasospasm is the typical finding. Unfortunately, vascular imaging may also be normal in the early phase of the illness.

Such patients must be admitted to hospital and monitored closely in the ICU or step-down floor. Because of altered cerebrovascular physiology, such patients are susceptible to infarcts in the setting of low blood pressure. Nimodipine and verapamil can be used. In rare cases with severe disease progression such as worsening infarction, intra-arterial vasodilation can also be used, although there is no large-scale data available to support its use.

132

• • • • •

A triad, autoimmune cause,
With impaired cognition,
Retinal/inner ear damage,
And corpus lesions in.

Hint #1

Often causes BRAO.

Hint #2

Look out for cannonballs and snowballs.

Susac Syndrome

First described by American neurologist John Susac in 1979, Susac syndrome (SS) is a rare autoimmune endotheliopathy causing microvascular damage to the brain, retina, and inner ear. As SS progresses it ultimately causes encephalopathy, branched retinal artery occlusion, and hearing loss. The underlying etiology is unknown; however anti-endothelial cell antibodies have been found in 30% of one cohort studied.

Rarely do all three clinical triad features present simultaneously at onset. The first signs of SS are usually of CNS impairment including memory loss/dementia, psychiatric symptoms, or seizure, and can precede vestibulocochlear and ophthalmologic findings by six months. Branched retinal artery occlusion most commonly presents as blurry vision or other visual field defects, and a hearing loss is usually unilateral and can progress to complete deafness.

Diagnosis typically requires dedicated retinal fluorescein angiography, audiometry, and brain MRI. Brain lesions are predominantly in white matter with lesions of the corpus callosum (informally known as *cannonball* or *snowball lesions*) being common and pathognomonic for SS. Cerebrospinal fluid analysis is nonspecific and often shows lymphocytic pleocytosis and elevated protein without oligoclonal banding.

Since this is a relatively rare disease, there are no large-scale studies of any specific treatment option. Most case reports, case series, and expert opinions suggest the use of high dose IV steroids. IVIG has also been used. The duration of treatment is variable and is determined by severity and progression of the disease. Overall, prognosis is considered good, and most patients show improvement in CNS and ophthalmologic symptoms with early aggressive treatment. Hearing loss usually does not recover. Delayed diagnosis and treatment can lead to irreversible cognitive impairment.

133

• • • • •

In those with seizures of full body,
Most 40 to post-teen,
Seize, then lungs and heart will fail,
A passing unforeseen.

Hint #1

The only treatment is prevention.

Hint#2

Most commonly associated with childhood-onset epilepsy.

Sudden Unexpected Death in Epilepsy (SUDEP)

Sudden unexpected death in epilepsy (SUDEP) is generally defined as the death of a patient with epilepsy determined not to be secondary to other known causes such as trauma, drowning, or status epilepticus with or without the evidence of recent seizure.

The cause of SUDEP is unknown, but the leading hypothesis is a postictal central apnea causing respiratory arrest, which in turn leads to a cardiac arrest. Postictal central apnea usually coincides with postictal generalized EEG suppression after a generalized tonic–clonic seizure. In addition, postictal obstructive apnea due to laryngeal spasm or neurogenic pulmonary edema could also lead to respiratory arrest. Hence, postictal generalized EEG suppression is considered a biomarker for SUDEP.

SUDEP mainly occurs between the ages of 25 and 45 in patients who have a history of refractory epilepsy with frequent generalized tonic–clonic seizures. The overall incidence of SUDEP is ~1 per 1000 person-years. This incidence is much higher in refractory epilepsies like Dravet syndrome, which has one of the highest rates of SUDEP ~10 per 1000 person-years.

The prevention of SUDEP depends on recognizing patients who are at risk. The highest risk occurs in younger patients who have refractory epilepsy with frequent generalized tonic–clonic seizures. The risk is significantly higher in patients who have sleep-related generalized tonic–clonic seizures and those without a bed partner. The main strategy to prevent SUDEP is to treat seizures aggressively.

134

• • • • •

Most common in athletes/soldiers,
Head impacts or post-blast,
Mood, cognition, movement change,
With tau in depths amassed.

Hint #1

Think "punch drunk."

Hint #2

Can only be diagnosed postmortem.

Chronic Traumatic Encephalopathy

First used in 1949, the term chronic traumatic encephalopathy (CTE) has been known by many names throughout medical history, including "punch drunk" in the 1920s, and dementia pugilistica coined in 1937 from the Latin work *pugil* meaning "boxer" or "fist." The cause of CTE remains heavily debated and is thought to be due to a combination of progressive microanatomical changes caused by repetitive closed-head injuries including direct impact from sporting collisions or blast exposures from military experience. Recent research has also proposed a genetic predisposition.

The prevalence of CTE is unknown as the diagnosis is made postmortem and studies have mainly analyzed those thought to be at highest risk, namely long-term athletes of contact sports and veterans with combat experience. Though studies have been published on the prevalence of postmortem diagnosis of CTE in professional sports players, these studies have been highly controversial and scrutinized over concern for bias.

The microanatomical changes associated with CTE are thought to be due to repeated acceleration, deceleration, and rotational forces acting on the brain in the cranial vault during an impact or blast. Histopathologically, these changes include but are not limited to tau-positive neurofibrillary tangle deposition at the depths of sulci and around small vessels (among other areas), and macroscopic changes such as pallor of the substantia nigra and locus coeruleus, as well as ventricular dilation.

Though the exact signs and symptoms of CTE, nor their prevalence, are known given the postmortem diagnosis required, these patients are generally thought to exhibit a combination of cognitive, behavioral, mood, and movement symptoms. These symptoms include impaired memory and executive function, anxiety, impulsivity, aggression, depression, mood lability, Parkinsonism, and ataxia, among many others. No anti-mortem testing has proven helpful in the diagnosis of CTE; however, research is ongoing on the role of gene ApoE and its possible contribution to tau deposition in these patients.

135

• • • • •

Born with dilated vessels on,
Half face who often seize,
Brain calcium deposits,
And hemiatrophies.

Hint #1

Also have leptomeningeal angiomatosis.

Hint#1

Unilateral glaucoma is common.

Sturge–Weber Syndrome

Sturge–Weber syndrome (SWS), also known as encephalofacial angiomatosis, is a neurocutaneous disorder named after English physician William Sturge and dermatologist Frederick Weber, who described its features in detail in 1869. Caused by congenital, nonhereditary (somatic) mosaic mutation of the gene GNAQ, this mutation disrupts vascular development, resulting in areas of abnormal vasculature on the face and intracranially and causing skin discoloration, leptomeningeal angiomatosis, and glaucoma.

The third most common neurocutaneous disease, SWS has no sex or race predominance. The cutaneous manifestations of SWS are usually facial and are also known as the "port-wine stain" or nevus flammeus. Port-wine stains are unilateral pink, red, or brown discolorations, typically found in the trigeminal nerve distribution, and are composed of dilated capillary malformations. Uncommonly, patients with SWS can have no port-wine stain. Leptomeningeal angiomatosis, an intracranial vascular anomaly is also found in the majority of those with SWS, usually located in the occipital and posterior parietal lobes, ipsilateral to the port-wine stain. These areas of abnormal vasculature cause focal impaired perfusion, resulting in seizures, stroke-like episodes, focal cerebral atrophy, and cerebral calcifications.

Glaucoma is also commonly seen in those with SWS and develops in infancy due to abnormal vascular formation (choroid hemangiomas) causing increased pressure within the eye. Most patients with SWS have some degree of developmental delay in childhood.

There is no cure for SWS. Epilepsy is the major neurological complication and requires treatment with anti-seizure medications. In refractory cases, surgery can also be considered. All experts recommend using low-dose aspirin from early childhood to prevent stroke-like events.

136

• • • • •

Encephalopathy, seizure,
And quadriparesis,
Slowly correcting serum salt,
Will help to avoid this.

Hint #1

Often seen outside the pons.

Hint #2

Highest risk in alcoholism and liver transplant.

Osmotic Demyelination Syndrome

Previously known as central pontine myelinolysis, osmotic demyelination syndrome (ODS) is an iatrogenic neurological syndrome first described in 1959 by neurologists Raymond Adams and Maurice Victor characterized by devastating CNS injury secondary to rapid serum sodium correction.

Historically, this syndrome was also separated into a subcategory called extrapontine myelinolysis in 1962 when lesions were also noted to be seen outside the pons. First thought to be a sequela of malnutrition and alcoholism, it wasn't until the 1980s that it was linked with rapid serum sodium correction.

Lesions are most commonly found in the basis pontis, sparing the pontine tegmentum; however, they can be found in many other areas of the brain, including but not limited to the cerebellum, basal ganglia, thalamus, internal and external capsules, cerebral cortex, hippocampus, midbrain, and medulla. Because most cases of ODS are thought to be clinically asymptomatic, frequency is unknown, but diagnosed cases are most common in males 30–60 years old with a history of either alcoholism or liver transplant.

Pathophysiology is poorly understood. It is proposed that patients with chronic hyponatremia have a lack of osmotically active osmolytes, which normally protect the neurons against swelling.

Clinical signs of ODS usually present in a biphasic manner. Encephalopathy with or without seizures is often the initial sign, and is usually seen while the patient is still hyponatremic. Then, after rapid correction to normonatremia, patients can develop flaccid tetraplegia, dysphasia, dysarthria, oculomotor abnormalities, severe changes in the level of consciousness, and in severe cases locked-in syndrome.

ODS is best prevented. Any patient with hyponatremia admitted to the hospital must not undergo a rapid correction. Sodium should be corrected by less than 8 meq/L in 24 hours in patients at high risk of ODS.

For patients who have signs and symptoms of ODS, serum sodium should be lowered again. But the prognosis is poor.

137

• • • • •

Nitrogen leaves solution,
Ascend, pressure gets light,
Paresthesias, limbs go weak,
As bubbles infarct white.

Hint #1

Found primarily in sea divers.

Hint #2

Disproportionately affects the spinal cord and inner ear.

Decompression Sickness (Caisson Disease/Bends)

Decompression sickness (DCS), also known as caisson disease, divers' disease, or *the bends* was first described by Irish alchemist Sir Robert Boyle in 1670 after seeing the effects of depressurizing a viper he had placed in a vacuum. Today, DCS is known as a multiorgan systemic condition in which nitrogen that is normally dissolved in tissues in a pressurized environment leaves the tissues in a gaseous state when the body enters a less pressurized environment. This is mostly seen in deep-sea divers experiencing high environmental pressures when diving, and then normal atmospheric pressure as they return to the water's surface. This condition has also been seen in pilots and astronauts.

In divers, DCS is seen after the inhaled mixed gases (such as a nitrogen and helium) from diving gear at high-pressure underwater depths are dissolved into connective tissue including skin, lymphatic tissue, muscle, and nervous tissue. During ascent from the high-pressure depths to a lower pressure environment, these dissolved mixed gases exit the tissue in gaseous form creating bubbles in the tissue. These bubbles not only create direct tissue damage with surrounding edema, but also endothelial damage (activating the coagulation cascade) causing blood vessel obstruction or vascular spasm, resulting in tissue ischemia. For unknown reasons, DCS has a male predominance.

Decompression sickness is divided into subtypes depending on the tissue involved. Type 1 involves extraneural tissue including skin, joints, muscles, and lymphatic system. The most common manifestation of DCS type 1 is joint pain (specifically shoulder pain), a condition informally known as "the bends," often co-occurring with skin mottling, rash, and pruritis. Type 2 DCS involves nervous tissue and only occurs in 10% to 15% of DCS cases. The most common areas affected by type 2 DCS are the spinal cord (specifically the thoracic spinal cord) as well as the inner ear. Symptoms of type 2 DCS include confusion, vertigo, and myelopathic signs such as weakness, numbness, paresthesia, and bowel and bladder dysfunction, which can progress if not treated effectively and quickly.

Diagnosis is clinical. The mainstay of treatment is recompression in a hyperbaric oxygen chamber.

138

• • • • •

Progressive increased tone in legs,
With weakness, reflex more,
Onset decades three to five—,
Spastin SPG4.

Hint #1

Almost never involves the arms.

Hint #2

A neurodegenerative disease.

Hereditary Spastic Paraplegia

Thought to be first described in 1880 by German neurologist Adolf Strumpell, hereditary spastic paraplegia (HSP) is a neurodegenerative disease resulting in degeneration of the spinal cord, primarily the corticospinal tract and dorsal columns. Unlike most other heritable neurological diseases, HSP can be inherited via almost any pattern, though most commonly autosomal dominant. Additionally, mutations in many genes have been implicated on at least 17 chromosomes and > 75 loci. The most common causal mutation is in the SPAST gene located on chromosome 2, producing the most common subtype, SPG4.

The pathophysiology of the HSP can vary widely; however, in general, clinical signs are produced primarily by the degeneration of the descending corticospinal tract and ascending dorsal columns with most severe degeneration occurring in the fibers traveling to the lower extremities and fibers of the fasciculus gracilis. Though anterior horn cells, dorsal roots ganglia, and peripheral nerves are usually spared, approximately 50% of cases do have some degree of spinocerebellar tract degeneration.

The age of onset of clinical signs of HSP varies widely depending on the subtype inherited, the inheritance pattern, and possible anticipation, though onset is most often between the second and fifth decade of life. Patients most often present with difficulty walking, stiffness, and weakness in the legs. On exam, patients with HSP have lower extremity spasticity, hyperreflexia, and upgoing toes on plantar response. Because of marked bilateral leg hypertonicity, those with HSP have a characteristic gait with leg circumduction and toe walking. Many patients also complain of sensory loss or paresthesias in the lower extremities, which typically presents later in disease progression. Muscle weakness is often most prominent in the hip, knee, and ankle flexors (iliopsoas, hamstrings, and tibialis anterior). Though anal sphincter

434

involvement is rare, urinary sphincter dysfunction is common and can produce urgency and incontinence in severe cases. Involvement of the arms is uncommon, and no involvement of the cranial nerves is present in HSP.

Diagnosis is clinical. MRI of spine and brain must be performed to rule out secondary causes of such a progressive syndrome. Other causes such as HIV, syphilis, HTLV-1 infection, vitamin B12 deficiency, and NMO must be ruled out. Final diagnosis is established with genetic testing.

There is no cure for HSP. Treatment is symptomatic, aimed at spasticity management with baclofen, tizanidine, and so on. Physical therapy is recommended as well.

139

● ● ● ● ●

Upper signs in two regions,
At least that oft' progress,
No lower signs or feeling loss,
Pre-central fibers less.

Hint #1

Only sporadic, not heritable.

Hint #2

Look for spasticity, weakness, and hyperreflexia.

Primary Lateral Sclerosis

Primary lateral sclerosis is a sporadic form of neurodegenerative motor neuron disease that affects almost exclusively upper motor neurons. The pathophysiology of PLS is similar to amyotrophic lateral sclerosis, and results in the degeneration of corticospinal tracts, though almost completely spares the lower motor neurons. Demographically, PLS symptoms usually begin in the fifth or sixth decade of life and have no significant sex predominance.

Most patients with PLS present with complaints of mild weakness, stiffness, clumsiness, and imbalance. On exam, key findings of PLS include hyperreflexia, spasticity, weakness, and the absence of lower motor neuron signs such as fasciculations and motor weakness. Sensation also remains intact. Weakness is often most prominent in extensor muscles of the upper extremity and the flexors of the lower extremity. Patients may also have bulbar symptoms including dysphagia and dysarthria, as well as signs of pseudobulbar affect and emotional lability. Cognition typically remains intact in those with PLS, though up to half report urinary urgency and frequency. Though the onset of symptoms can present asymmetrically, progression is usually symmetrical, eventually resulting in spastic tetraplegia.

Imaging with MRI is indistinguishable from ALS and can show atrophy of motor and premotor cortex or T2 hyperintensity of the corticospinal tract. The utility of EMG is primarily to rule out other possible diagnoses such as amyotrophic lateral sclerosis.

Treatment of PLS is supportive with symptomatic management of spasticity and physical therapy. Prognosis is better than classic ALS.

140

• • • • •

A clot most often septic caused,
And pain as eye will swell,
Sixth nerve stops working, followed by,
The third and fourth as well.

Hint #1

Beware facial infections or procedures.

Hint #2

Consider treating with antibiotics and anticoagulation.

439

Cavernous Sinus Thrombosis

Cavernous sinus thrombosis (CST) is a neurological emergency characterized by thrombosis of the cavernous sinus resulting in pain and multiple cranial neuropathies. There is minimal epidemiological data on CST; however those with facial infections such as sinusitis, dental or periorbital infections, or recent facial or dental procedures are at the highest risk. The most common cause of septic thrombosis is a *Staphylococcus aureus* infection of the middle face. Non-septic causes of CST include thrombophilic disorders such as factor V Leiden and other heritable thrombophilias, as well as acquired disorders such as antiphospholipid syndrome.

The cavernous sinuses are a pair of dural venous sinuses next to the sella turcica and the pituitary gland. Each sinus contains the internal carotid artery surrounded by a peri-arterial sympathetic plexus. Other cranial nerves in the cavernous sinus include abducens (CN VI), which is located immediately next to the internal carotid artery. Other nerves include oculomotor (CNIII), trochlear (CNIV), and ophthalmic and maxillary divisions (V1 and V2) of the trigeminal nerve.

Cavernous sinus syndrome presents with headache, retroorbital pain, chemosis, proptosis, and any combination of cranial neuropathies as mentioned above. This clinical presentation must prompt emergent investigation with a brain MRI, MRI orbits with and without contrast, and MR venography as well. If the presence of cavernous sinus thrombosis is confirmed, treatment with therapeutic anticoagulation is recommended. In cases of septic cavernous sinus thrombosis, antibiotics must be initiated as well.

141

• • • • •

Different regions, single nerve,
That hurt, go weak, and swell,
Asymmetric autoimmune,
And stop recruiting well.

Hint #1

Foot drop then wrist drop.

Hint #2

One nerve at a time.

Mononeuritis Multiplex

Mononeuritis multiplex (MNM), also known as mononeuropathy multiplex, is a pattern of neuropathy that affects multiple nerves, but one at a time in different anatomical locations, rather than group nerves. The nerves affected, by definition, cannot be explained by the dysfunction of a single nerve root or plexus.

Several diseases and conditions can cause MNM including vasculitides such as polyarteritis nodosa and granulomatosis with polyangiitis, connective tissue diseases such as systemic lupus erythematosus and rheumatoid arthritis, endocrine diseases such as diabetes mellitus and autoimmune inflammatory diseases such as amyloidosis, sarcoidosis, and Sjogren syndrome. Additionally, infections such as Lyme disease and leprosy can cause MNM.

Those with MNM often present with acute onset localized severe painful dysesthesias and sensory loss, followed by focal motor weakness in the distribution of that nerve, most often presenting asymmetrically in the distal extremities as foot drop, wrist drop, or other focal weaknesses. For example, these patients might first present with forearm pain and wrist drop followed shortly thereafter by severe leg pain and ankle drop. On exam, patients often have preserved tendon reflexes and some degree of allodynia. The most commonly affected nerves include the peroneal nerve (most common), sural nerve, tibial nerve, ulnar nerve, median nerve, and radial nerve.

The diagnosis relies on detailed clinical history and a thorough neuromuscular examination. Supporting information can be obtained by nerve conduction studies and needle electromyography. Once a clinical and/or electrodiagnostic diagnosis of MNM is established, further tests to identify a specific etiology must be performed. This could include testing for autoimmune conditions

442

and systemic vasculitis. A nerve biopsy can also be performed to confirm the diagnosis of vasculitis affecting a nerve.

The mainstay of treatment is steroids. For long-term treatment, steroid sparing agents such as rituximab, azathioprine, or cyclophosphamide can be used.

142

. . . . .

Monophasic, nonprogressive,
At birth or before,
Hypoxia or trauma cause,
Ataxic and tone more.

Hint #1

Risk factors include low birth weight and prematurity.

Hint #2

Typically diagnosed in early childhood.

Cerebral Palsy

Cerebral palsy (CP) is a neurological syndrome caused by injury to the developing brain during the perinatal period that produces permanent nonprogressive neurological dysfunction. Risk factors for CP include prematurity, low birth weight, multiple gestations, infertility treatments, infection during pregnancy, Rh incompatibility, and perinatal toxin/drug exposure, among others. Though most cases of CP are caused by prenatal or natal cerebral injury (termed congenital CP) from hypoxic–ischemic injury, the most common cause of postnatal CP is traumatic brain injury, near-drowning, and meningitis.

Many infants determined to be at high risk are screened and subsequently diagnosed early; however, approximately half of those with CP aren't diagnosed until early childhood when medical care is sought for delayed milestones or atypical neuromotor development. Though CP is a monophasic condition, clinical features may become more prominent and evolve over time through childhood as other physical abilities develop.

Cerebral palsy can present with a wide variety of neurological signs, with the most common clinical findings being persistence of primitive reflexes, spasticity, ataxia, and truncal hypotonia. The most common clinical phenotype is spastic diplegia that often portends a good prognosis; though many have spastic tetraplegia, more commonly portending a poorer prognosis for functional independence. Extrapyramidal signs are also common in CP and include dystonia, choreoathetosis, or dyskinesia. Epilepsy is a commonly occurring comorbidity as well.

On neuroimaging, specifically on MRI, periventricular leukomalacia, with severe cases showing multicystic cortical encephalomalacia, can be seen.

Treatment is supportive and symptomatic. Epilepsy is treated with anti-seizure medications. Spasticity is treated with baclofen and physical therapy is recommended. Children often have special needs as far as education is concerned because of intellectual disability.

143

• • • • •

In those cortically blind, both sides,
Anterior intact,
Confabulate their surroundings,
As if they see they act.

Hint #1

In bilateral occipital lobe lesions.

Hint #2

A type of visual anosagnosia.

Anton Syndrome

Anton syndrome (AS), also called Anton–Babinski syndrome, is a rare form of visual anosognosia seen in patients with lesions of bilateral occipital lobes (primary visual cortices). It is thought that AS was first unknowingly described by Roman philosopher and politician Seneca in AD 63, who wrote in his *Moral Letters of Lucilius* about his wife's slave who had become acutely blind but could not appreciate her blindness. Though another case would be described by French Renaissance writer Michel de Montaigne in the sixteenth century, this condition would not be described by a physician until 1864 when Austrian neurologist and psychiatrist Gabriel Anton described the case of "Ursula M," who denied her objective blindness. The term anosognosia was later coined by François Babinski in 1914, referring to a patient's unawareness of his/her neurological or physical deficits.

The exact neurophysiology of AS is unknown; however, there are two proposed theories. One theory postulates a disconnection between the conscious awareness system of the frontal and parietal lobes that monitors and integrates the sensory input, and the visual cortex of the occipital lobe that would visualize a deficit, resulting in the lack of awareness of a patient's visual deficits. Another theory postulates that deficits in vision lead to false-positive feedback from the visual cortex. The cause of blindness in AS is most commonly cerebral infarction; however, it can also include trauma, hemorrhage, posterior reversible encephalopathy syndrome, among many others.

On evaluation, patients with Anton syndrome have complete cortical blindness; however, they deny their blindness and confabulate things in their visual field. When confronted about their blindness, these patients often continue to deny their deficits.

There is no specific treatment for Anton syndrome. The prognosis depends upon the reversibility of the underlying cause of blindness.

144

• • • • •

Most often from hyperextend,
Most common in c-spine,
Weakness in arms is worse than legs,
Some numb, vibration fine.

Hint #1

Affects medial fibers first.

Hint #2

Still not sure? Ask the man in a barrel.

Central Cord Syndrome

Central cord syndrome (CCS) is the most common form of incomplete spinal cord injury, typically resulting from impingement of the cervical spinal cord after hyperextension injury. Though CCS can present at any age because of trauma to the cervical spine such as from a fall forward or direct impact to the neck, it most commonly presents in those over 50 with underlying degenerative disc disease which can narrow the spinal canal, predisposing these individuals to spinal cord injury in the case of hyperextension.

As the name suggests, the affected structures are in the central part of the spinal cord, including the medial portions of the descending lateral corticospinal tracts and ascending spinothalamic tracts. All white matter tracts have a somatotopic organization. For both corticospinal tracts and spinothalamic tracts, arm fibers are more medial than the leg fibers; hence the weakness and sensory loss in CCS mainly affect bilateral upper extremities with relative sparing of lower extremities. This pattern of weakness is also referred to as cruciate paralysis and it has high localizing value to high cervical spinal cord.

Clinically, these patients present with neck pain after hyperextension injury with either isolated bilateral upper extremity weakness or upper extremity disproportionate to lower extremity weakness. Core muscles of the torso are also often affected to a lesser degree than the upper extremities, causing an axial and postural weakness. Those with CCS also often experience a "cape-like" pattern of decreased pain and temperature sensation over the upper back, arms, and to a lesser degree through the torso. *Sacral sparing* is a typical finding in those with CCS, as sacral sensation is often preserved. Though dorsal columns can be affected, vibration and proprioceptive sense usually remain intact. These patients also often experience bladder dysfunction such as urinary retention. The relatively unique motor presentation of CCS is informally known as "man in a barrel syndrome."

This is a neurological emergency and warrants emergent investigation with MRI of the C-spine. Emergent neurosurgical intervention is warranted to decrease the risk of irreversible damage.

145

• • • • •

Fluid-filled and central pos'd,
Cavity, most spine-c,
Arms lose pain and reflexes,
Segmental atrophy.

Hint #1

Can be within or outside canal.

Hint #2

Usually congenital, and found incidentally.

Syrinx/Syringomyelia/Hydromyelia

Strictly speaking, there are slight neuroanatomical and neuro-pathological differences in syringomyelia and hydromyelia, but given their similar symptomology and difficulty to differentiate on neuroimaging, they are grouped using the general term "syrinx."

Syringomyelia is a cavitary lesion in the central portion of the parenchyma of the spinal cord, adjacent to the central canal, and thus not lined by ependymal cells. This is caused by a cystic dissection of the ependymal lining of the central canal that results in CSF accumulation within the spinal cord parenchyma, not within the central canal. Hydromyelia is a dilation within the central canal of the spinal cord caused by CSF accumulation, and thus lined by ependymal cells. The term syringohydromyelia is used when the components of both hydromyelia and syringomye-lia are thought to be present.

Most cases of syrinx are congenital and found concomitant with myelomenignoceles, type I and II Chiari malformations, Dandy-Walker malformations, and other neuroaxis malformations. The minority of cases of syrinx are acquired and caused by trauma in the setting of spinal cord injury. Rarely a syrinx is caused by nontraumatic injury to the spinal cord, such as sequela of spinal cord tumor, spinal cord infarction, infection, or inflammatory lesions.

Though most cases are found incidentally on neuroimaging, the clinical presentation of those with syrinx varies widely depending on its location in the neuroaxis and causal conditions. Common signs and symptoms include bilateral loss of pain and temperature sensation at the level of the lesion resulting from injury to the crossing spinothalamic tract fibers. Most cases of syringomyelia occur at the level of the cervical cord, resulting in sensory changes in bilateral arms.

As the area of CSF accumulation grows, injury to the descending corticospinal tract fibers and alpha motor neurons can occur, resulting in weakness. In cases of congenital causes of syrinx such as Chiari malformation, these findings are often concomitant with headache, bulbar dysfunction (dysphagia, hoarseness), visual disturbance, and cerebellar dysfunction.

Neuroimaging with MRI is most sensitive and will show a central dilation and CSF accumulation within or adjacent to the central canal of the spinal cord. Treatment is mainly surgical.

146

• • • • •

In those that temporally spike,
Change personality,
Hyper-religious, write too much,
Low sexuality.

Geschwind Syndrome

Geschwind syndrome (GS) was first described in 1975 by American neurologists Norman Geschwind and Stephen Waxman as a behavioral syndrome consisting of hyper-religiosity, hyposexuality, hypergraphia, and irritability. Though GS has classically been described in patients with temporal lobe epilepsy, it has also been reported in cases of frontotemporal dementia, temporal strokes, and hippocampal atrophy. Interestingly, most cases are associated with a nondominant lobe pathology.

These clinical findings are constant and typically progressive over time; and in the case of temporal lobe epilepsy, they are not considered ictal phenomena but interictal traits. Though the exact pathophysiology is unknown, recent studies in the right temporal lobe variant of frontotemporal lobar degeneration have reported similar behavioral changes, further suggesting pathological localization to the nondominant temporal lobe.

Clinically, those with this constellation of behavioral symptoms will often present with exaggerated religious or philosophical concerns, compulsive documentation, abnormally decreased sexuality, and interpersonal stubbornness. The diagnostic workup for these individuals should include EEG, brain MRI, and neuropsychiatric assessment.

There is no specific treatment. It is important to identify the underlying cause such as temporal lobe epilepsy and treat it accordingly.

147

• • • • •

Neonatal/infants in,
Tonic spasm, burst suppress,
In sleep and wake refractory,
To others will progress.

Hint #1

Can be seen in the first weeks of life.

Hint #2

Most commonly associated with brain malformations.

Ohtahara Syndrome

Named after Japanese child neurologist Shunsuke Ohtahara, who first described its characteristics in 1976, Ohtahara syndrome (OS) is a rare form of early infantile developmental epileptic encephalopathy. A majority of cases of OS are associated with underlying structural brain abnormalities such as hemimegalencephaly, porencephaly, cortical dysplasias, and neuronal migration disorders. Several genetic mutations have also been associated with OS, most common being STXBP1, followed by KCNQ2. Many primary metabolic disorders are also associated with OS, such as nonketotic hyperglycinemia and other amino and organic acid disorders. Ohtahara syndrome affects males and females equally.

Those with OS typically begin having generalized or lateralized tonic seizures (spasms) within the first few weeks to months of life that can present in isolation or in clusters, and last up to 10 seconds. Spasms have no association with sleep cycle. After the development of spasms, other seizure semiologies can develop, including generalized tonic–clonic seizures and focal motor seizures. The development of myoclonic seizures is uncommon and can help differentiate OS from other epilepsy syndromes.

Electroencephalographic analysis of patients with OS shows a generalized burst suppression pattern in both wakefulness and sleep, with spasms correlating with EEG bursts.

Ohtahara syndrome is an electroclinical syndrome with multiple potential etiologies. If these children survive, the syndrome can evolve into other forms of developmental epileptic encephalopathies such as West syndrome and Lennox–Gastaut syndrome.

Treatment requires anti-seizure medications, but seizures are often refractory to treatment. If the underlying cause is structural (e.g., hemimegalencephaly), epilepsy surgery must be considered and could significantly reduce the seizure burden and improve development. If a specific genetic mutation is found, precision treatment can be used. For example, KCNQ2 mutation-related Ohtahara syndrome will likely respond well to sodium channel blockers.

.

148

• • • • •

For those with frontal damage and,
Most often on side-right,
Excessively make puns/bad jokes,
Understand jokes cannot quite.

Hint #1

Hopefully you speak German.

Hint #2

They often miss the punchlines of others.

Witzelsucht

First described by German neurologist Herman Oppenheim in 1898, the term "witzelsucht" comes from the German words "witz" meaning *joke* and "sucht" meaning *addiction* or *obsession*. This term is used to describe the pathological and inappropriate joking, pun-making, and/or childish excitement, most commonly seen in patients with lesions of the right frontal lobe, specifically the right orbitofrontal region. Witzelsucht has been reported in patients with right (or bilateral) frontal lobe brain tumors, infections, trauma, cerebral infarcts and hemorrhages, and neurodegenerative diseases such as frontotemporal lobe dementia.

The compulsive joke-making these patients exhibit is typically socially and age-inappropriate; however, many of these patients remain age-appropriate on cognitive testing. Interestingly, these patients are often unable to understand the humor in jokes made by others. More specifically, patients with witzelsucht have difficulty connecting the punchline of the jokes of others with the storyline of the joke; however, they are able to find humor in slapstick comedy.

The neurophysiology of witzelsucht is assumed to be due to disinhibition produced by orbitofrontal cortex injury with right frontal lesions leaving these individuals more sensitive to simple and slapstick comedy and with impaired comprehension of complex storylines.

149

· · · · ·

Same side eye cannot look outward,
And face will droop side same,
Other has no vibration sense,
Feels numb and strength is lame.

Hint #1

Consider the brainstem.

Hint #2

Look out for lacunes.

Foville Syndrome/Inferior Medial Pontine Stroke

First described by French neurologist and psychiatrist Achille-Louis Foville in 1858, Foville syndrome (FS) describes the syndrome of neurological sequela occurring after lesion to the inferior medial pons. Most commonly, FS presents due to lacunar infarct of the pons, but it can also occur in the setting of hemorrhage, tumor, or inflammatory lesion. In the case of lacunar infarction, this is secondary to occlusion of the paramedian pontine branches of the basilar artery.

Because of the high concentration of the cranial nerve nuclei and long tracts that travel medially through the pons, FS presents with a highly variable mix of cranial nerve palsies and long tract signs.

The classic presentation is ipsilateral horizontal conjugate gaze palsy caused by lesion of the abducens nucleus with ipsilateral lower motor neuron-type facial palsy because of the lesion of the facial nerve (as it wraps around the abducens nucleus). In addition, patients could also have INO because of lesion of the MLF. The combination of the conjugate horizontal gaze palsy and INO is referred to as one and a half syndrome. This, in combination with ipsilateral facial palsy is referred to as eight and a half syndrome. The involvement of the descending corticospinal tract in ventral pons can cause contralateral weakness. The lesion of medial lemniscus can produce contralateral sensory deficit as well.

If the lesion is more ventral, then the presentation will be slightly different – ipsilateral abduction paresis (abducens nerve injury) and contralateral weakness (because of corticospinal tract injury). The facial nerve will be preserved because it exits more laterally. This syndrome is known as Raymond syndrome.

150

• • • • •

Diplopia worse same-side gaze,
And tongue will bend same side,
Just two palsied nerves involved,
Clival lesion reside.

Hint #1

Involved nerves add up to 18.

Hint #2

Most caused by tumor.

Godtfredsen Syndrome

First described by Danish ophthalmologist Eric Godtfredsen in 1946, Godtfredsen syndrome (GS) is a rare clinical syndrome characterized by a combination of abducens nerve and hypoglossal nerve palsies.

Both of these are pure motor nerves and exit medially from the brainstem. The abducens nerve enters the prepontine cistern, whereas the hypoglossal nerve enters the premedullary nerve. Both of these cisterns are situated against the clivus bone. Large pathologies affecting the clivus such as clival chordoma, nasopharyngeal cancer, and plasmacytoma can present with this unique combination of cranial nerve palsies.

Patients presenting with GS have horizontal diplopia because of abduction paresis resulting from abducens nerve injury and tongue weakness due to hypoglossal nerve injury.

This unique clinical syndrome should prompt a brain MRI with and without contrast to evaluate for tumors invading the clivus. Treatment will depend upon the underlying cause.

Index

1. Subdural Hematoma 2
2. REM Sleep Behavior Disorder 6
3. West Syndrome 8
4. Epidural Hematoma 10
5. Locked-in Syndrome 12
6. Restless Leg Syndrome 14
7. Amaurosis Fugax 18
8. Vascular Dementia 20
9. Neurosyphilis 24
10. Transverse Myelitis 28
11. Duchenne Muscular Dystrophy 32
12. Subacute Combined Degeneration 36
13. Dermatomyositis 40
14. Wernicke-Korsakoff Syndrome 42
15. Lambert Eaton Myasthenic Syndrome 44
16. Absence Epilepsy 46
17. Acute Inflammatory Demyelinating Polyradiculoneuropathy 48
18. Migraine Headache 52
19. Progressive Supranuclear Palsy 56
20. Myasthenia Gravis 60
21. Subarachnoid Hemorrhage 64
22. Amyotrophic Lateral Sclerosis 68
23. Essential Tremor 72
24. Polymyositis 74
25. Huntington Disease 76
26. Creutzfeldt-Jakob disease 80
27. CNS Toxoplasmosis 84
28. Autism Spectrum Disorder 86
29. Botulism 88
30. Large Right Middle Cerebral Artery Territory Cerebral Infarction 92
31. Alzheimer's Disease 96
32. Meningioma 100
33. Dravet Syndrome 102
34. Large Left Middle Cerebral Artery Territory Cerebral Infarction 106
35. Stiff Person Syndrome 110
36. Cluster Headache 112
37. HSV-1 Encephalitis 116
38. Trigeminal Neuralgia 118
39. Cerebral Amyloid Angiopathy 120
40. Charcot-Marie Tooth 122
41. Multiple Sclerosis 126
42. Transient Global Amnesia 130
43. Temporal Arteritis 134
44. Autoimmune Encephalitis 138
45. Inclusion Body Myositis 142
46. Medulloblastoma 144
47. Lateral Medullary Syndrome 148
48. Arteriovenous Malformation 152
49. Normal Pressure Hydrocephalus 154
50. Fungal Meningitis 158
51. Tetanus 162
52. Cerebral Venous Sinus Thrombosis 166
53. Idiopathic Intracranial Hypertension 168
54. Neuromyelitis Optica Spectrum Disorder 172
55. Neurocysticercosis 176
56. Spinal Muscular Atrophy 180
57. Juvenile Myoclonic Epilepsy 184
58. Glioblastoma Multiforme 186
59. Multiple System Atrophy 190
60. Neuroleptic Malignant Syndrome 194
61. Posterior Reversible Encephalopathy Syndrome 196

62. Epidural Abscess 198
63. Pituitary Adenoma 202
64. Central Nervous System Lymphoma 206
65. Lennox–Gastaut Syndrome 210
66. Neurosarcoidosis 212
67. Miller Fisher Syndrome 216
68. Generalized Tonic-Clonic seizure 218
69. Short-Lasting Unilateral Neuralgiform Attacks with Conjunctival Injection and Tearing Syndrome 220
70. Intracranial Hypotension Headache 222
71. Psychogenic Nonepileptic Seizures 224
72. Parkinson Disease 226
73. Hemicrania Continua 230
74. Carotid or Vertebral Dissection 232
75. Acute Motor Neuron Neuropathy 236
76. Chronic Inflammatory Demyelinating Polyradiculoneuropathy 240
77. Subacute Sclerosing Panencephalitis 244
78. Progressive Multifocal Leukoencephalopathy 248
79. Friedreich Ataxia 252
80. Disseminated Lyme disease (neuroborreliosis) 254
81. Meige Syndrome 258
82. Acute Disseminated Encephalomyelitis 260
83. Corticobasal Degeneration 262
84. Psychogenic Tremor 266
85. Frontotemporal Dementia 268
86. Ependymoma 272
87. Tourette Syndrome 274
88. Myotonic Dystrophy 278
89. Benedikt Syndrome (Medial/Ventral Midbrain Infarction) 282
90. Oligodendroglioma 284

91. Gerstmann–Straussler–Scheinker Syndrome 286
92. Fatal Familial Insomnia 288
93. Mitochondrial Encephalopathy, Lactic Acidosis, and Stroke-Like Episodes Syndrome 290
94. Merrf Syndrome 292
95. Concussion 294
96. Rasmussen Syndrome/Encephalitis 298
97. Ataxia–Telangiectasia 300
98. Panayiotopoulos Syndrome 304
99. Unruptured Intracranial Aneurysm 306
100. Cerebral Autosomal Dominant (or Recessive) Arteriopathy with Subcortical Infarcts and Leukoencephalopathy (CADASIL/CARASIL) 310
101. Tardive Dyskinesia 314
102. Lance–Adams Syndrome 318
103. Orthostatic Tremor 320
104. Doose Syndrome 322
105. Cauda Equina Syndrome 326
106. Brown-Sequard Syndrome 328
107. Bell's Palsy 332
108. Hemiplegic Migraine 336
109. Vertebral Disc Herniation/Radiculopathy 340
110. Charles Bonnet Syndrome 344
111. One and a Half Syndrome 348
112. Tolosa–Hunt Syndrome 350
113. Internuclear Ophthalmoplegia 354
114. Benign Paroxysmal Positional Vertigo 358
115. Vestibular Neuritis/Labyrinthitis 362
116. Neurofibromatosis 1 366
117. Tuberous Sclerosis 368
118. Ménière Disease 372
119. Catatonia 374
120. Spinal Cord Infarction 378
121. Kluver–Bucy Syndrome 382
122. Diabetic Amyotrophy 384
123. Marchiafava-Bignami Disease 388

472

124. Opsoclonus–Myoclonus–Ataxia Syndrome 390
125. Balint Syndrome 394
126. Parsonage–Turner Syndrome/ Brachial Plexitis 396
127. Hypokalemic Periodic Paralysis 398
128. Holmes–Adie Syndrome 402
129. Transient Ischemic Attack 404
130. Postural Orthostatic Tachycardia Syndrome 408
131. Reversible Cerebral Vasoconstriction Syndrome 412
132. Susac Syndrome 416
133. Sudden Unexpected Death in Epilepsy 418
134. Chronic Traumatic Encephalopathy 420
135. Sturge–Weber Syndrome 424
136. Osmotic Demyelination Syndrome 426
137. Decompression Sickness (Caisson Disease/Bends) 430
138. Hereditary Spastic Paraplegia 434
139. Primary Lateral Sclerosis 438
140. Cavernous Sinus Thrombosis 440
141. Mononeuritis Multiplex 442
142. Cerebral Palsy 446
143. Anton Syndrome 450
144. Central Cord Syndrome 452
145. Syrinx/Syringomyelia/ Hydromyelia 456
146. Geschwind Syndrome 460
147. Ohtahara Syndrome 462
148. Witzelsucht 466
149. Foville Syndrome/Inferior Medial Pontine Stroke 468
150. Godtfredsen Syndrome 470

For EU product safety concerns, contact us at Calle de José Abascal, 56–1°,
28003 Madrid, Spain or eugpsr@cambridge.org.

www.ingramcontent.com/pod-product-compliance
Ingram Content Group UK Ltd.
Pitfield, Milton Keynes, MK11 3LW, UK
UKHW021957061225
465726UK00011B/294